A–Z of Abdominal Radiology

A–Z of Abdominal Radiology

Gabriel Conder, MRCP, FRCR

Consultant Radiologist,
Northwick Park and Central Middlesex Hospitals, North West London
Hospitals NHS Trust, London

John Rendle, FRCS (Eng), FRCR

Consultant Radiologist
Mayday University Hospital, Mayday Healthcare NHS Trust, Croydon

Sarah Kidd, MRCP, FRCR

Specialist Registrar in Radiology
St. Mary's Hospital, Imperial College Healthcare NHS Trust, London

Rakesh R. Misra, BSc (Hons), FRCS (Eng.), FRCR

Consultant Radiologist
Wycombe Hospital, Buckinghamshire Hospital NHS Trust, High Wycombe

Series Editor

R. R. Misra

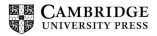

CAMBRIDGE
UNIVERSITY PRESS

CAMBRIDGE UNIVERSITY PRESS
Cambridge, New York, Melbourne, Madrid, Cape Town, Singapore, São Paulo, Delhi

Cambridge University Press
The Edinburgh Building, Cambridge CB2 8RU, UK

Published in the United States of America by Cambridge University Press, New York

www.cambridge.org
Information on this title: www.cambridge.org/9780521700146

First published 2009

Printed in the United Kingdom at the University Press, Cambridge

A catalogue record for this publication is available from the British Library

ISBN 978-0-521-70014-6 paperback

To my beautiful wife Rachel, and four inspirational
children – Rohan, Ela, Krishan and Maya.   **R. R. M.**

To my mother and father – very different people, but
both inspirational.   **G. C.**

CONTENTS

ACKNOWLEDGEMENTS

I would like to thank my consultant colleagues Carolyn Charlesworth, Philip Cadman, Richard Hughes, Dinuke Warakaulle, Eric Woo and Vipin Uthappa for their help in sourcing so many of the varied images needed for this book. Your time and effort is greatly appreciated.

Thanks to my good friend Miles Berry, who helped to conceive the idea for this book in a Parisian bistro in 2001.

R. R. M.

The authors would also like to thank Professor W. Gedroyc and Drs Jon Ord and David Burling for contributing several important images.

PREFACE

The *A-to-Z of Abdominal Radiology* is a valuable addition to the *A-to-Z of Radiology* series, continuing the theme of concise introductions to specific fields of radiology. The text is concisely laid out, following a similar format to the other title in this series, using a bullet point format to allow rapid assimilation of relevant facts. The text is richly illustrated with images from modern scanners.

The book will be a useful aid to medical students, radiographers, surgical trainees, physicians and emergency doctors who wish to gain a greater understanding of abdominal and pelvic imaging and how it can improve their clinical practice. Radiology trainees will also find this a helpful aide-mémoire to consolidate their knowledge.

G. C.
J. R.
S. K.
R. R. M.

ABBREVIATIONS

^{99m}Tc	technetium-99m
AAA	Abdominal aortic aneurysm
ACE	Angiotensin-converting-enzyme
AIDS	Acquired immunodeficiency syndrome
AP	Antero-posterior
ARDS	Adult respiratory distress syndrome
ATLS	Advanced trauma life support
AXR	Abdominal X-ray
CA19-9	Carbohydrate antigen 19-9
CECT	Contrast-enhanced computed tomography
CNS	Central nervous system
CT	Computed tomography
CXR	Chest X-ray
ERCP	Endoscopic retrograde cholangiopancreatography
FDG	Fluorodeoxyglucose
FIGO	Federation international de gynaecologie et obstetrique
FNH	Focal nodular hyperplasia
GI	Gastrointestinal
Gy	Gray
HCC	Hepatocellular carcinoma
HD	Hodgkin's disease
HU	Hounsfield unit
IUCD	Intrauterine contraceptive device
IV	Intravenous
IVC	Inferior vena cava
IVU	Intravenous urogram
KUB	Kidney–ureter–bladder
LBO	Large-bowel obstruction
LIF	Left iliac fossa
LUQ	Left upper quadrant
MALT	Mucosa-associated lymphoid tissue
MIBG	Meta-iodobenzylguanidine
MR	Magnetic resonance
MRCP	Magnetic resonance cholangiopancreatography
MRI	Magnetic resonance imaging
NECT	Non-enhanced CT
NHL	Non-Hodgkin lymphoma

NM	Nuclear medicine
PET	Positron emission tomography
PID	Pelvic inflammatory disease
PTC	Percutaneous trans-hepatic cholangiogram
RAS	Renal artery stenosis
RIF	Right iliac fossa
RLQ	Right lower quadrant
RPF	Retroperitoneal fibrosis
RTA	Road traffic accident
RUQ	Right upper quadrant
SBO	Small-bowel obstruction
T1W	T1 weighted
T2W	T2 weighted
TA	Trans-abdominal
TB	Tuberculosis
TCC	Transitional cell carcinoma
TIPS	Transjugular intrahepatic porto-systemic shunt
TURBT	Transurethral resection of bladder tumour
TURP	Transurethral resection of prostate
TV	Transvaginal
UC	Ulcerative colitis
UK	United Kingdom
US	Ultrasound
USS	Ultrasound scan
VIP	Vasoactive intestinal polypeptide
WBC	White blood cell count

A–Z OF ABDOMINAL RADIOLOGY

Abdominal trauma

Clinical characteristics

- A general discussion, followed by organ-specific summaries, is given below.
- Abdominal trauma is managed as part of general trauma under the ATLS (advanced trauma life support) algorithm, where basic care of airway, breathing and circulation is followed by a secondary survey and simultaneous management.
- Abdominal trauma is usually divided into **blunt** and **penetrating** trauma.

Penetrating trauma

- Generally managed by surgical exploration and repair. Surgical repair may be primary or secondary (delayed) according to a multitude of factors, including degree of contamination, time since injury and general health of the patient.
- Where the patient is haemodynamically unstable, with signs of obvious massive intra-abdominal haemorrhage, many of the investigations below are suspended, and the patient is managed surgically on an emergency basis with coexistent haemodynamic monitoring and management.
- If the patient is haemodynamically stable, the usual radiological investigation is a contrast-enhanced computed tomography (CECT) scan. This is usually performed following a radiographic primary survey (lateral cervical spine, chest and pelvis radiographs).
- It is now generally considered that diagnostic peritoneal lavage is rarely indicated and has been superseded by CECT.
- Emergency ultrasound (US) of the abdomen and pelvis is sometimes performed and may be of use in determining the presence and location of intra-abdominopelvic blood. Vascularity of abdominal viscera (e.g. the kidneys) can also be assessed. US may also be used to monitor patients who are being managed conservatively. However, CECT is considered superior in the context of acute abdominal trauma.

Blunt trauma to the spleen

- Spleen is the most commonly injured solid intra-abdominal organ.
- Blunt trauma is the most common cause.
- Often (40%) associated with lower rib fractures and left renal injury.
- In 20% of patients with left rib fractures, there is a concomitant splenic injury.

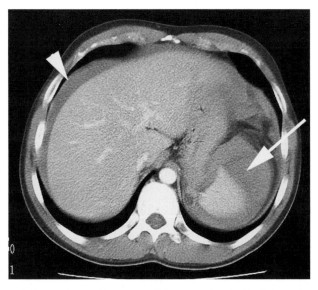

Rupture of the spleen. Rupture of the anterior half of the spleen caused by blunt trauma in falling from a horse. Haemorrhage is seen within the splenic bed (arrow) along with free blood around the liver (arrowhead).

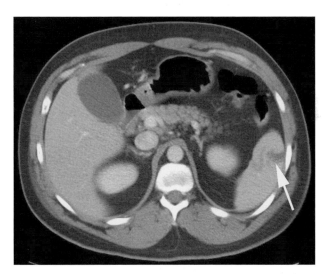

Splenic laceration (arrow).

- 25% of patients with left renal injuries also have splenic injuries.
- Damage ranges from subcapsular haematoma to total splenic laceration, potentially leading to exsanguination.

Radiological features

- **Abdominal X-ray (AXR):**
  - Poor sensitivity in identifying both the site and presence of intra-abdominal haemorrhage.
  - May show associated fractures, displaced air-filled bowel caused by intra-abdominal blood or free air from associated bowel perforation.
- **CECT:**
  - In nearly all cases of abdominal trauma, a CECT of the abdomen and pelvis is performed to ensure adequate coverage of injuries.
  - Mottled splenic parenchymal enhancement may represent contusion. **NB.** The spleen in the arterial phase of a CECT may normally appear mottled.
  - Splenic fracture may present as complete separation of unenhancing splenic fragments.
  - Subcapsular haematoma is shown by a crescentic region of low attenuation compressing normal parenchyma.
  - Intracapsular haematoma is demonstrated by a hypodense inhomogeneous region within the spleen.
  - Splenic laceration is revealed as a hypoattenuating line connecting opposite visceral surfaces. Associated with perisplenic fluid.
  - Multiple lacerations represent a shattered spleen.
  - Disruption of the splenic capsule with high-density fluid within abdomen represents splenic rupture with free intraperitoneal haemorrhage.

Complications

- Splenic pseudocyst formation.
- Delayed rupture – up to 10 days later.
- Infected subcapsular haematoma.
- Splenic artery pseudoaneurysm.

Blunt trauma to the liver

- Second most frequently injured intra-abdominal organ.
- Associated with splenic injury in 45%.
- Right lobe more frequently injured.
- When left lobe is involved, there may be associated injury to the duodenum, pancreas and transverse colon.

Radiological features

- **AXR:**
  - Increased density in RUQ, displacement of neighbouring organs, e.g. right kidney displaced downwards and medially.

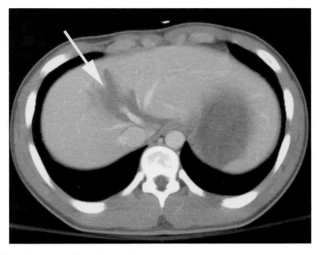

Large liver laceration (arrow).

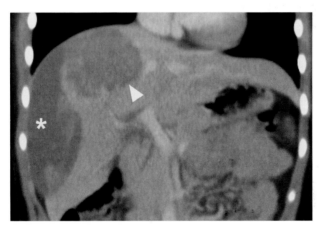

Liver haematoma. Large haematoma within the superior aspect of the right lobe of liver (arrowhead) with an additional subcapsular haematoma (asterisk).

- **CECT:**
  - Subcapsular haematoma – hypoattenuating lenticular configuration, usually resolves in 6–8 weeks and generally managed conservatively.
  - Hepatic laceration – irregular linear branching, single or multiple stellate configurations of low density relative to enhancing parenchyma.
  - Focal hepatic devascularisation – focal hypodense wedge lesion extending to liver surface.
  - Active haemorrhage – focal hyperdense area.
  - Hepatic necrosis – intrahepatic or subcapsular gas.

Complications

- Occur in up to 20%.
- Haemobilia.
- Pseudoaneurysm/arteriovenous fistula formation.
- Biloma.
- Infection/necrosis.
- Delayed hepatic rupture – unusual.

Blunt trauma to the kidneys

- Occurs in 10% of blunt abdominal injury.
- Often caused by a direct blow (80%).
- Usually caused by laceration by lower ribs or devascularisation of the renal pedicle in acceleration–deceleration injuries.
- Associated with other abdominal organ injury in 20%.
- Almost always presents with some degree of haematuria (over 95%).
- Main exception is with renal pedicle injuries, where 25% have no haematuria due to devascularisation of kidney.
- Not usually accompanied by lower renal tract injury.
- Four degrees of injury, ranging from contusion and corticomedullary laceration (grade I) to renal pedicle avulsion (grade IV).

Radiological features

- **AXR:** Plain film findings commonly seen in renal trauma include:
  - Absent psoas shadow.
  - Enlarged/distorted kidney and pelvicalyceal system (following administration of IV contrast).
  - Fractures of the 10th, 11th and 12th ribs.
  - Fractures of the transverse processes of the 1st, 2nd or 3rd lumbar vertebra.
  - Scoliosis, concave towards the injured side, due to associated muscle spasm.
  - Localised small-bowel/colonic ileus.
- **US:**
  - May show devascularisation, renal swelling from a diffuse haematoma, peri- or pararenal haematoma, renal laceration or ureteric obstruction from a ureteric clot.
- **CECT:**
  - Renal contusion – focal areas of decreased contrast enhancement or striated nephrogram.
  - Renal laceration – irregular linear hypodense parenchymal areas.
  - Renal fracture – laceration connecting two cortical surfaces.
  - Shattered kidney – multiple separated renal fragments.
  - Subcapsular haematoma – crescentic superficial hypodense area.
  - Wedge infarction – wedge-shaped perfusion defect.

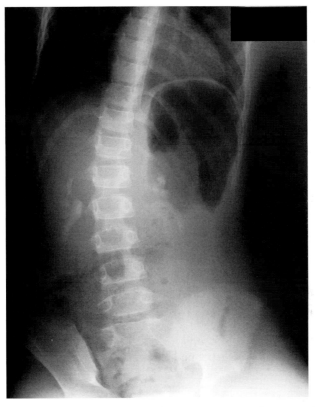

Closed blunt right renal trauma. There is asymmetry between the two renal outlines, with distortion of the left pelvicalyceal system and left renal outline. In addition there is a scoliosis of the thoracolumbar spine, concave towards the injured side, and a localised ileus of the splenic flexure. Normal contrast excretion seen from the right kidney.

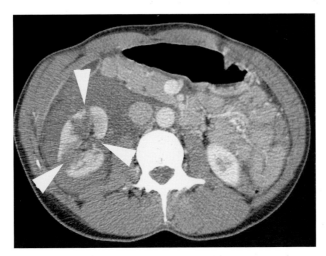

Kidney trauma. Multiple fractures of the right kidney (arrowheads) caused by blunt trauma from a kick by a horse. Extensive surrounding perinephric haemorrhage.

- Renal vein thrombosis – persistent delayed nephrogram.
- Delayed scans are also often performed to check for a ureteric leak.

Blunt trauma to pancreas

- Usually caused by compression against the vertebral column; often associated with seat belt compression injuries.
- Usually associated with upper abdominal visceral injury.
- Graded from minor contusion and capsular haematoma (grade I) to severe devascularising crush injury (grade IV).
- Usually damage occurs at most vulnerable segment of pancreas: the junction of the body and tail.

Radiological features

- **CECT:**
  - Laceration – area of intrapancreatic low attenuation, often difficult to see.
  - Direct evidence of haemorrhage – fluid around superior mesenteric artery and pancreas.
  - Indirect evidence – thickening of anterior pararenal fascia.
- Often requires delayed scans to exclude/monitor complications of pancreatitis and devascularised pancreas.

Complications

- Post-traumatic pancreatitis, with:
  - peripancreatic fat stranding
  - diffuse or focal pancreatic enlargement
  - irregular pancreatic contour.
- Splenic vessel fistula or arterial pseudoaneurysm.
- Pancreatic abscess.
- Pancreatic pseudocyst.

Blunt Trauma to the gastrointestinal tract

- The proximal jejunum is most commonly affected, followed by the duodenum and ascending colon at the ileocaecal valve region. The descending colon is only rarely involved.

Radiological features

- **CECT:**
  - Appearances range from mesenteric or intramural haematoma to frank colonic laceration and perforation.

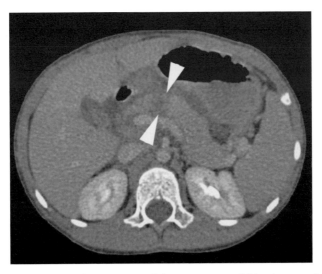

Pancreatic trauma. Laceration of the pancreas within the proximal body (arrowheads).

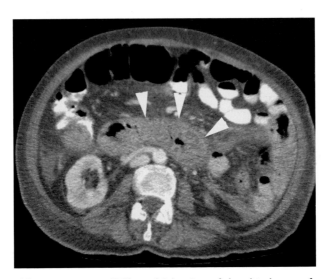

Duodenal haematoma. Diffuse thickening of the third part of duodenum secondary to a post-traumatic duodenal haematoma (arrowheads).

- Subtle helpful signs include streaky hyperdense mesentery, sentinel clot sign adjacent to local bowel injury, and hyperdense enhancement of bowel wall in delayed venous phase caused by mesenteric vascular damage.

Less-common abdominal trauma injuries

- Gallbladder.
- Ureter.
- Stomach.
- Adrenals.

Trauma to the bladder

Aetiology and frequency

The probability of bladder injury varies according to the degree of bladder distension; a full bladder is more likely to be injured than an empty one.

- Approximately 10–25% of patients with a pelvic fracture also have urethral trauma. Conversely, 10–29% of patients with posterior urethral disruption have an associated bladder rupture.
- **External trauma**: 80%.
  - Blunt injury: 60–85%:
    - road traffic accident (RTA), 85%.
    - fall, 10%.
    - assault, 5%.
  - Penetrating trauma: 15–40%:
    - gunshot wound, 85%.
    - stabbing, 15%.
- **Iatrogenic**: 15%.
  - Includes gynaecological (post-hysterectomy), urological (after transurethral resection of prostate (TURP) or bladder tumour (TURBT)) and orthopaedic (post-fixation of pelvic fractures) procedures.
- **Intoxication**: 4%.
- **Spontaneous**: <1%.

Classification of bladder rupture

- Extraperitoneal rupture: 50–75%.
- Intraperitoneal rupture: 25–45%.
  - Incidence higher in children because of the predominantly intra-abdominal location of the bladder prior to puberty.
  - The bladder descends into the pelvis usually by the age of 20 years.
- Combined extraperitoneal and intraperitoneal rupture: 5–10%.

Extraperitoneal bladder rupture

- Traumatic extraperitoneal ruptures are usually associated with pelvic fractures in up to 90% of patients. Conversely, approximately 10% of patients with pelvic fractures also have significant bladder injuries.

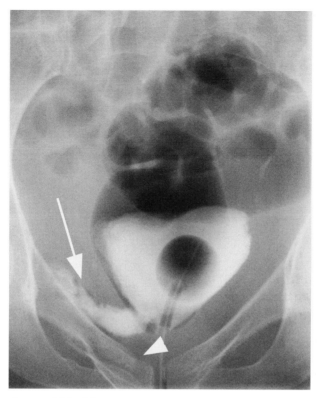

Extraperitoneal bladder rupture following a fall. Cystogram demonstrates extravasation of contrast in to the right hemipelvis, tracking along the peritoneal reflection (arrow). Note the fracture of the right superior pubic ramus (arrowhead).

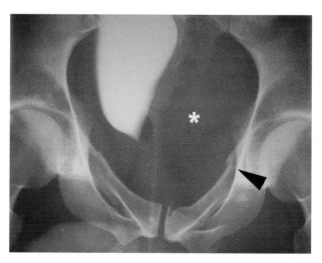

Large left pelvic haematoma (asterisk) secondary to a pelvic fracture (arrowhead). Cystogram reveals that the bladder is elevated and compressed to the right, producing a so-called 'tear drop' shape to the bladder.

- Results from the shearing force of the deforming bony pelvic ring, which causes a 'burst' injury.
- Bony fragments may also cause direct laceration of the bladder and the degree of bladder injury is directly related to the severity of the fracture.

Intraperitoneal bladder rupture

- Occurs as the result of a direct blow to a distended urinary bladder. The resulting increased intravesical pressure causes a horizontal tear along the intraperitoneal portion of the bladder wall. This type of injury is common amongst alcoholic patients or those sustaining blunt trauma following a RTA.

Clinical characteristics

- Clinical signs of bladder injury are relatively non-specific; however, a triad of symptoms is often present:
  - gross haematuria
  - suprapubic pain or tenderness
  - difficulty or inability to void.
- Abdominal examination may reveal distension, guarding or rebound tenderness.
- Absent bowel sounds and signs of peritoneal irritation indicate a possible intraperitoneal bladder rupture.
- If blood is present at the urethral meatus, suspect a urethral injury.

Radiological features

- **CT:**
  - Often the first test performed in patients with blunt abdominal trauma.
  - Provides information on the status of the pelvic organs and bony pelvis.
  - **CT cystography:**
    - The most sensitive test for evaluating a bladder perforation.
    - Contrast is instilled into the bladder via a urethral catheter (or suprapubic catheter if contraindicated) followed by an abdominopelvic CT scan.
    - Intraperitoneal and extraperitoneal nature of a rupture can be accurately assessed.
- **Cystogram:**
  - Standard imaging for a suspected bladder injury.
    - Consists of an initial plain radiograph of the kidney–ureter–bladder (KUB).
    - Followed by AP and oblique views of the contrast-filled bladder.
    - Further AP film obtained after drainage.

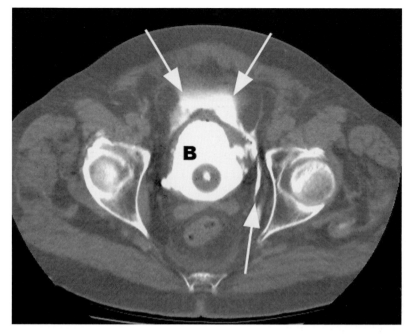

Extraperitoneal bladder perforation following a transurethral resection of a bladder tumour. This CT cystogram clearly demonstrates contrast extravasation into the perivesical soft tissues (arrows). Note the presence of several bladder diverticula and a Foley balloon catheter within the bladder (B).

- **Extraperitoneal rupture:**
  - Contrast extravasation around the base of the bladder is confined to the perivesical space. The bladder may assume a tear-drop shape from compression by a pelvic hematoma.
  - With more complex injuries contrast may extend into the thigh, penis, perineum or anterior abdominal wall.
- **Intraperitoneal rupture:**
  - Contrast extravasation into the peritoneal cavity, often outlining loops of bowel and the paracolic gutters.
- **Combination of intra- and extraperitoneal rupture:**
  - Contrast outlines the abdominal viscera and perivesical space.

Abscesses within the abdomen

Peritoneal abcesses

Clinical characteristics

- Accumulation of collections of pus in the peritoneal spaces.
- Subphrenic abcesses are usually secondary to surgery.
- Paracolic abcesses are usually local to their cause, such as diverticulitis, appendicitis or anastomotic failure.
- They present with raised inflammatory markers, swinging pyrexia, pain and malaise.

Radiological features

- **AXR:** abscesses are often of soft tissue density and, therefore, difficult to see. The presence of gas makes the identification easier. The finding of gas pockets outside the bowel lumen, particularly if its appearance does not change over time, is highly suggestive. A subphrenic gas–fluid level on an erect chest X-ray (CXR) or erect AXR is suggestive of a collection in this region.
- **USS:** an effective test for abdominal collections, being sensitive for fluid collections or gas–fluid collections. It can also be used for guided percutaneous drainage. Occasionally deep collections may be obscured by overlying bowel gas.
- **CECT:** very sensitive for collections and may identify those obscured on US. CT guidance can be utilised for percutaneous drainage.
- **NM:** using [111]indium labelled white cell scans are very sensitive for detecting peritoneal abscesses but are infrequently used as the use of CT increases.

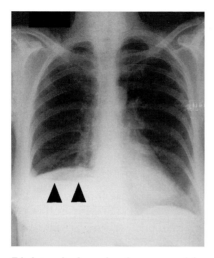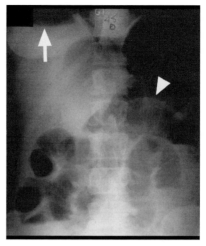

Right subphrenic abscess and free air. Air–fluid level below the right hemidiaphragm (black arrowhead and white arrow) and a Riggler's sign (white arrowhead).

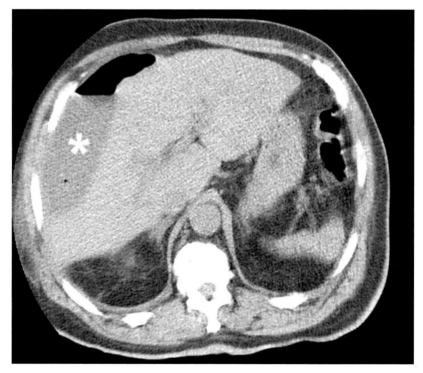

Large hepatic subcapsular abscess containing air (asterisk). Note the effacement of the adjacent right lobe of liver, confirming the subcapsular position.

Perirenal and renal abscesses

Clinical characteristics

- A complication of renal infection (see Pyelonephritis).
- 80% of cases result from ascending infection; may be related to obstruction.
- Haematogenous spread causes 20%.
- Urine culture may be negative.
- A renal abscess that extends through the renal capsule becomes a perinephric abscess.

Radiological features

- **AXR:** provides clues as to the presence of a perinephric abscess. These include loss of psoas shadow, focal mass seen in the renal outline, displacement of the renal outline and gas in the renal bed. Calculi may also be seen.
- **USS:** a hypo- or anechoic irregular mass, ± gas bubbles, ± perinephric extension, may be demonstrated. Guided drainage can be performed.
- **Intravenous urogram (IVU):** a renal abscess may distort the pelvic-alyceal system, but any mass lesion, such as a simple cyst, can have this effect and hence an IVU is poorly specific.
- **CT:** may demonstrate a mass lesion with a low-density centre, and an enhancing wall. Perinephric spread will be demonstrated and causal factors, such as calculi, identified. Guided drainage can be performed.
- **NM:** inflammatory change in the renal bed may be demonstrated with a radiolabelled white cell scan.

Hepatic abscesses

Clinical characteristics

- Most commonly secondary to biliary sepsis.
- Other causes include sepsis arriving via the portal venous system (i.e. portal pyaemia, e.g. appendicitis), direct spread, indwelling arterial lines and direct contamination associated with trauma.
- Pyogenic organisms (88%), amoebic (10%), fungal (2%).
- Presentation may include pyrexia, vomiting, abdominal pain, jaundice and positive blood cultures.

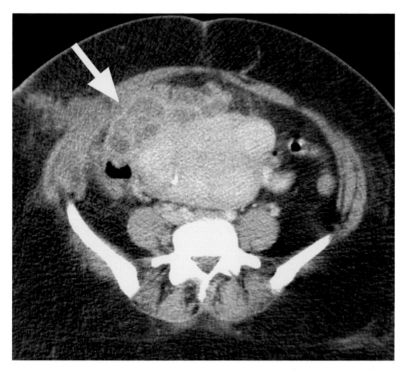

Post-appendicectomy abscess. Note the complex multiloculated collection deep to the incision (arrow).

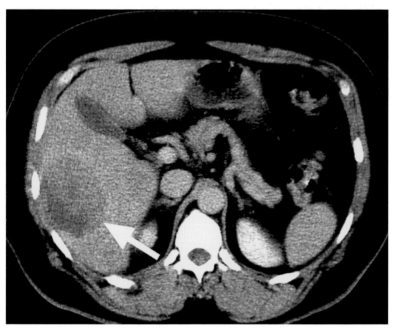

Liver abscess. Heterogeneous collection within the right lobe of the liver (arrow).

Radiological features

- **USS:** may demonstrate an irregular collection containing thick debris ± trough enhancement, ± gas bubbles. Amoebic abscesses rarely contain gas and may demonstrate internal septations. US-guided drainage may be performed.
- **CT:** heterogeneous hypodense lesion with mural enhancement.

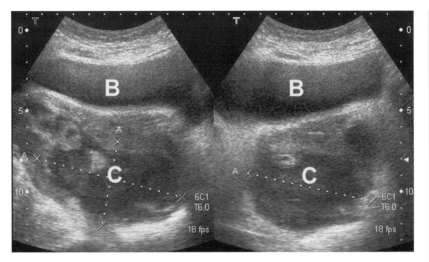

Pelvic abscess. Complex collection (C) deep within the pelvis. B, bladder.

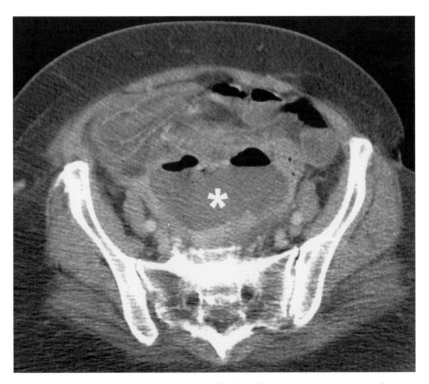

Pelvic abscess (same patient). large fluid collection, containing pockets of air, deep within the pelvis (asterisk).

Achalasia

Clinical characteristics

- This is a motility disorder that results in failure of relaxation of the lower oesophageal sphincter.
- The sphincter will only relax when the hydrostatic pressure of the column of food, or liquid, in the oesophagus exceeds that in the stomach, more usually in the erect position.
- May be of primary or secondary aetiology; most commonly primary. Secondary achalasia occurs rarely in diseases such as malignancy, diabetes mellitus and Chagas' disease.
- Peak age of incidence is 20–40 years, but it has been diagnosed in children.
- Most common presentation is dysphagia. Patients may also complain of retrosternal chest pain from oesophageal distension and effortless regurgitation of undigested food.
- Complications include aspiration pneumonia and an increased incidence of oesophageal cancer.

Radiological features

- **Plain X ray:**
  - An air–fluid level may be seen within the dilated oesphagus on the chest radiograph.
  - A small or absent gastric bubble may be present on the abdominal radiograph, but this is non-specific and generally an AXR is not helpful.
- **Barium studies:**
  - The barium swallow is the radiological investigation of choice.
  - Findings include:
    - Failure of oesophageal peristalsis to clear the oesphagus of barium.
    - Failure of relaxation of the lower oesophageal sphincter.
    - Poorly coordinated peristaltic activity.
    - Oesophageal dilatation is a late feature.
    - Narrowing of the oesophagus at the lower sphincter resulting in characteristic 'bird's beak' tapering.
  - The barium study may be normal, particularly in the early stages of the disease.
  - Radiological findings should be confirmed by endoscopy and manometry and, if necessary, biopsies to exclude a secondary cause such as malignancy, or to exclude malignancy as a complication of long-standing achalasia.

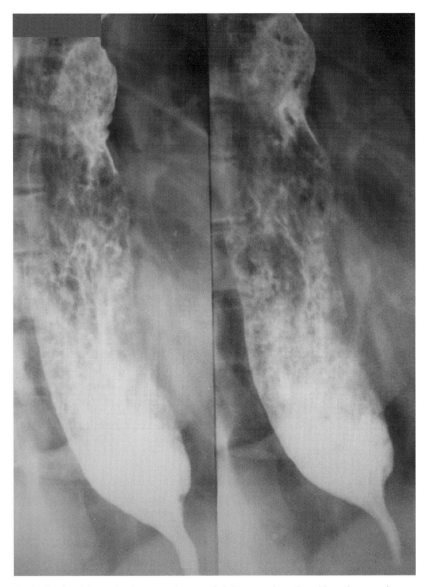

Achalasia. Note the large volume of debris within the dilated oesophagus and the characteristic 'bird's beak' tapering at the lower sphincter.

- The radiological findings characteristic of achalasia, with normal mano-metric readings, are a feature of pseudoachalasia, a condition that occurs in tumours of the distal oesophagus or lower oesophageal sphincter.
- **CT:** demonstrates the dilated oesophagus but this is non-specific.
- **NM, MRI and USS:** these modalities do not have a role in the diagnosis of achalasia.

Adnexal masses

Clinical characteristics

- In anatomical terms the adnexa are considered to include the uterine (fallopian) tubes and ovaries. Each ovary lies posterolaterally on either side of the uterus, attached to the broad ligaments by its own mesentery, the mesovarium, and to the uterus by the ovarian ligament. The fallopian tubes lie in the superior aspect of the broad ligament. Each tube is approximately 10 cm long and from the uterus runs posteriorly, laterally and then inferiorly.
- The presentation of ovarian disease includes pain, menstrual irregularities, infertility, dyspareunia or abdominal distension, or it may be an incidental finding.
- Ovarian pathology can be divided into the following categories:
  - Benign physiological cysts:
    - follicular cysts
    - corpus luteal cysts.
  - Benign mixed solid/cystic lesions
    - mucinous cystadenoma
    - serous cystadenoma
    - teratoma/dermoid
    - endometriosis.
  - Benign solid tumours
    - granulosa cell tumour
    - fibroma
    - Brenner tumour.
- Malignancy: primary/secondary.
- Pathology of the uterine tubes can be caused by pelvic inflammatory disease (PID), ectopic pregnancy or rarely carcinoma.
- Acute PID will present with pain and fever and possibly a palpable mass in the adnexa.
- The chronic form is often asymptomatic and may only be diagnosed during investigation for infertility or pelvic pain.
- Non-gynaecological causes of adnexal masses include an appendix mass or diverticular disease.
- Imaging features of ovarian neoplasias are rarely definitively diagnostic.

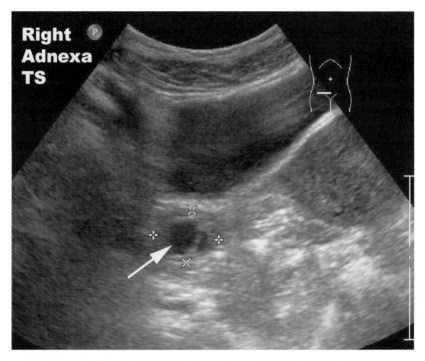

Ovarian cyst. Follicular cyst within the right ovary (arrow).

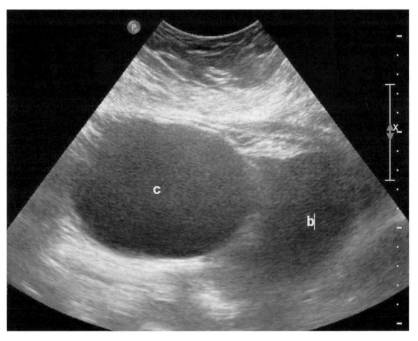

Large anechoic right ovarian cyst (c) indenting the superior aspect of the bladder (b).

Radiological features

- **AXR:** plain films do not have a role in the diagnosis of adnexal pathology. Any abnormality on an AXR is likely to be an incidental finding (e.g. calcification within an ovarian dermoid cyst).
- **Contrast studies:**
  - The hysterosalpingogram is used to demonstrate the uterine tubes using x-ray screening following the instillation of iodinated contrast into the uterine cavity via the cervical os.
  - It forms part of the investigation of infertility to assess tubal patency.
  - The ovaries will not be visible on x-ray screening.
- **USS:**
  - Trans-abdominal (TA) and transvaginal (TV) US is the modality of choice for initial gynaecological imaging.
  - Because of the anatomy of the adnexa, the positions of the ovaries can be very variable and dependent on the degree of distension of the urinary bladder. Pregnancy also affects laxity of the ligaments.
  - The TA US is usually done with a full bladder and TV US with an empty bladder.
  - For both TA and TV US, a good anatomical landmark for the ovaries is the internal iliac artery.
  - Ovarian cysts are very common and are usually considered normal unless >20–25 mm in diameter (cut off varies between institutions) or the patient is prepubertal, pregnant or postmenopausal.
  - Cysts >20–25 mm in women of reproductive age are usually rescanned at a different stage of the menstrual cycle, for example 2 weeks later, to document their physiological nature.
  - Malignant ovarian masses are usually more complex than benign lesions and US is used to assess ovarian morphology.
  - Indicators of malignancy include larger size, thick cyst wall, internal septations, solid components and mixed echogenicity cyst fluid. Blood flow assessment and pulsed Doppler are also of use.
  - The normal non-dilated fallopian tube is not visible ultrasonically but can be seen following the instillation of an US micro-bubble contrast medium via the cervical os. This technique, known as hysterosalpingo-contrast sonography (HyCoSy), is used as an alternative to the hystero-salpingogram to assess tubal patency.
  - The abnormal dilated tube (a hydrosalpinx), in chronic PID for example, appears as a serpiginous structure in the pelvis.
  - An important adnexal mass is that of ectopic pregnancy, of which 97% are tubal. The US findings in ectopic pregnancy are absence of a uterine pregnancy, an adnexal mass and free intraperitoneal fluid.

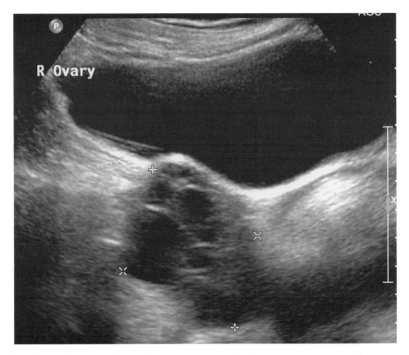

Ovarian abscess. Complex multiseptated right ovarian mass with eccentric wall thickening (callipers).

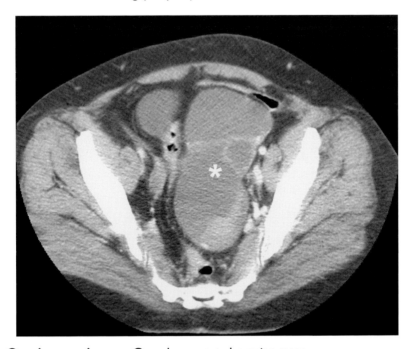

Ovarian carcinoma. Complex septated ovarian mass (asterisk) containing a large enhancing solid component posteriorly.

- **CT:**
  - CT is of some use in diagnosing adnexal masses but US and MRI provide more internal detail, owing to better soft tissue differentiation, without the radiation dose.
  - CT is sensitive for fat or calcification within a mass, for example in a dermoid tumour.
- **MRI:**
  - Can provide excellent resolution of the pelvis and is very useful in the assessment of gynaecological pathologies.
  - Used with fat suppression, it is sensitive for the fat seen in dermoid tumours.
  - Sensitivity for different blood breakdown products means MRI is sensitive for endometrial deposits where fluid–fluid levels, caused by haemorrhage of different ages, are seen within endometriotic cysts.
- MRI features that suggest malignancy in an ovarian cyst:
  - size >4cm.
  - soft tissue, non-fatty mural nodules.
  - large soft tissue component.
  - mural or septal thickness of >3mm.
  - mural or septal irregularity.
  - metastatic deposits or direct spread.
  - presence of ascites and peritoneal nodules.

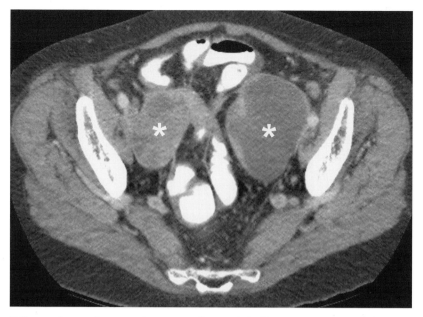

Bilateral ovarian carcinomata (asterisks). The right ovarian mass is predominantly solid while the left is largely cystic with eccentric wall thickening.

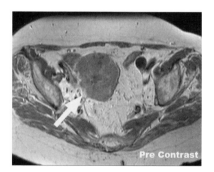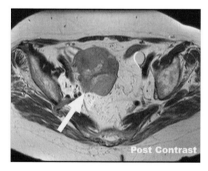

Right ovarian carcinoma: axial T1W MRI pre- and postcontrast. Large enhancing solid right adnexal mass (arrow).

Adrenal masses

Clinical characteristics

- The adrenal glands have a 'Y' configuration with an anteromedial body and two posterior limbs.
- The right adrenal gland lies between the right crus of the diaphragm and IVC at the level of the upper pole of the kidney. The left adrenal extends from the upper pole of the left kidney almost to the hilum. It lies in front of the left crus of the diaphragm.
- Usually the limbs are 3–6 mm thick and the width of the entire gland is <1 cm.
- The adrenal cortex produces glucocorticoids (cortisol), mineralocorticoids (aldosterone) and androgens. The adrenal medulla produces adrenaline and noradrenaline.

Causes of adrenal masses

- **Functional:**
  - adenoma causing Conn's or Cushing's syndrome.
  - phaeochromocytoma.
  - adrenal carcinoma.
- **Malignant:**
  - metastases.
  - carcinoma.
  - lymphoma.
  - neuroblastoma.
- **Benign:**
  - non-functioning adenoma.
  - angiomyolipoma.
  - cyst.
  - haemorrhage.

- The most common neoplasms are adenomata and metastastic disease. A common indication for adrenal imaging is to differentiate between these.
- The presentation of adrenal masses depends upon whether the mass is functional or not.
- Non-functioning tumours such as adenoma are usually an incidental finding when the patient is imaged for another reason.

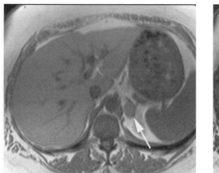
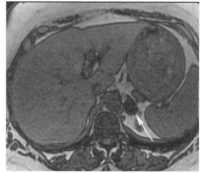

Adrenal adenoma. 'In-phase' (A) and 'out-of-phase' (B) MRI confirms loss of signal in a lipid-rich left adrenal adenoma (arrows) on the out-of-phase image compared with the corresponding in-phase imaging.

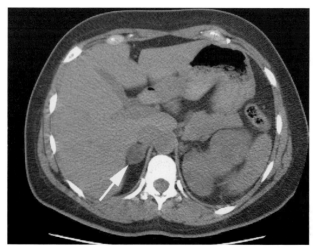

Adrenal adenoma. Low-density non-functioning right adrenal adenoma (arrow).

- With a functional adenoma, the presentation varies with the type of hormone being produced in excess.
  - Conn's syndrome is caused by excess aldosterone and results in hypertension, hypokalaemia and alkalosis.
  - Cushing's syndrome is caused by excess glucocorticoid and results in myopathy, osteoporosis, water retention, obesity of the trunk, head and neck, hypertension, predisposition to infection, easy bruising, and hyperglycaemia.
  - Phaeochromocytoma is a neuroendocrine tumour that secretes catecholamines, resulting in hypertension, cardiomyopathy, weight loss and hyperglycaemia. The 'rule of 10s' applies to phaeochromocytoma: 10% are adrenal, 10% are bilateral, 10% are malignant.

Radiological features

Adrenal adenomas versus metastatic deposits

- **USS:**
  - Although the adult adrenal glands may be visualised on US, it is usually the surrounding fat that is visible.
  - The adrenals appear hypoechoic relative to the fat but may only be seen when abnormally enlarged.
  - By contrast the neonatal adrenal is readily seen because of its larger size relative to the other intra-abdominal organs, smaller patient size and less retroperitoneal fat.
  - Adrenal masses usually appear hypoechoic, but haemorrhage or necrosis results in a heterogeneous appearance.
  - It is important to differentiate adrenal masses from masses arising from the adjacent liver, spleen, kidneys and pancreas.
- **CT:**
  - CT is a well-established modality for investigating adrenal masses and uses the fact that the majority of adenomata have high lipid content.
  - A non-contrast CT is performed and the CT number (Hounsfield units (HU)) of the mass measured. If the HU is ≤ 10 it is considered to be a benign adenoma on the basis of its fat content.
  - If the HU is > 10, an enhanced 80-s and a 15-min delayed postcontrast CT are obtained, and the enhancement washout calculated. The washout is a measure of the percentage decrease between the enhanced and delayed images.
  - A large decrease is a high percentage washout and a small decrease is a low percentage washout.
  - If the enhancement washout is $> 50\%$, the diagnosis of a benign lipid-poor adenoma is made.
  - If the washout is $< 50\%$, the mass is considered indeterminate, and a biopsy may be necessary to make a diagnosis, particularly in a patient with a new extra-adrenal primary neoplasm.
  - Metastatic deposits are usually larger and more heterogeneous than adenomata and do not have intracellular fat. Even in patients with known malignant primaries, half of all adrenal masses will be benign.

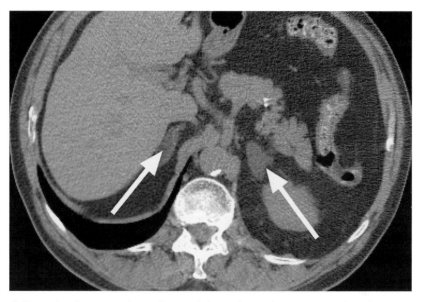

Adrenal adenoma. Low-density bilateral non-functioning adrenal adenomata (arrows).

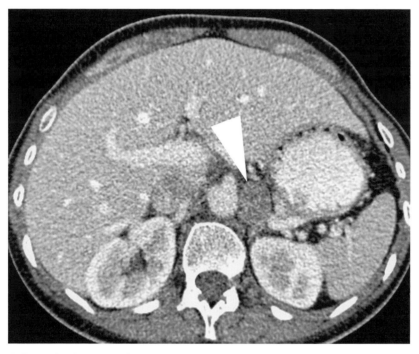

Adrenal adenoma. Low-density functioning left adrenal adenoma, producing Conn's syndrome (arrowhead).

- **MRI:**
  - MRI also makes use of the lipid content of adenomata.
  - In-phase and out-of-phase (also known as chemical shift) imaging demonstrates a loss of signal in a lipid-rich adenoma, on the out-of-phase image compared with the corresponding in-phase imaging.
  - A metastatic deposit does not demonstrate this loss of signal.
  - Chemical shift imaging only provides the same information about an adrenal mass as CT by identifying the lipid–rich subset of adenomata.

Intervention

- Adrenal venous sampling can be performed to identify whether the abnormal hormone production is unilateral or bilateral: most commonly in primary hyperaldosteronism (Conn's syndrome).

Phaeochromocytoma

Radiological features

- **US:**
  - Phaeochromocytoma may be visible as a well-defined mass, which may be solid or cystic to variable degrees.
  - Echogenicity will be variable.
- **CT:**
  - Phaeochromocytomas are usually large with a homogeneous density, although larger masses may appear heterogeneous owing to haemorrhage or necrosis.
  - Show strong contrast enhancement.
  - Some authors believe that IV contrast administration may precipitate a hypertensive crisis and recommend alpha and beta blockade prior to IV contrast.
- **MRI:**
  - Phaeochromocytoma have very high signal intensity on T_2-weighted (T2W) images, higher than adenoma or metastasis, and usually iso- or hypointense on T_1-weighted (T1W) imaging.
  - Strong enhancement which may be heterogeneous depending on the degree of cystic change.

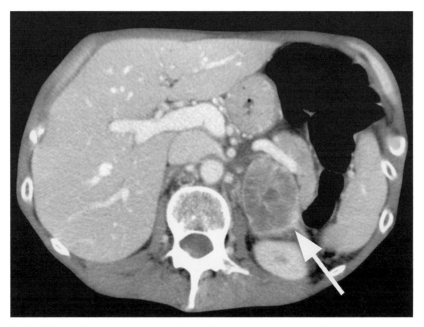

Left phaeochromocytoma. Large heterogeneously enhancing
left adrenal mass.

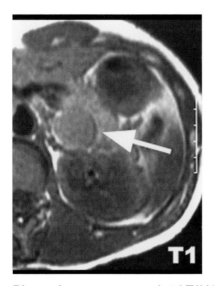

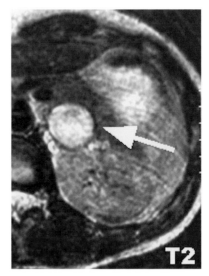

Phaeochromocytoma: Axial T1W and T2W MRI. The lesion is
isointense on T1W and markedly hyperintense on T2W.

- **NM:**
  - NM has a role in the diagnosis of phaeochromocytoma. ^{131}I-MIBG and ^{123}I-MIBG are concentrated in the sympathomedullary system and focal uptake is seen in phaeochromocytoma. Whole-body imaging will demonstrate extra–adrenal tumours.

Adrenocortical carcinoma

- A rare carcinoma of the 4th to 7th decade.
- May present with Cushing's syndrome if hyperfunctioning.
- Other presentations include pain and a mass.
- Usually >5 cm in diameter at presentation.
- One-third show calcification.
- Can invade adjacent structures including the IVC.
- May metastasise to nodes, bones and lungs.

Radiological features

- **USS:**
- Tumour necrosis and haemorrhage result in heterogeneous echogenicity.
- **CT:**
- Central area is of low density owing to necrosis.
- May be calcification and areas of haemorrhage.
- Irregular peripheral enhancement following contrast.
- **MRI:**
- The mix of haemorrhage and necrosis results in heterogeneous signal on both T1W and T2W imaging.
- Irregular peripheral enhancement.

Myelolipoma

- A benign tumour composed of haematopoietic tissue and fat. Unlike adenomas, the fat is discrete fat rather than intracellular.
- Can present with painful haemorrhage.

A

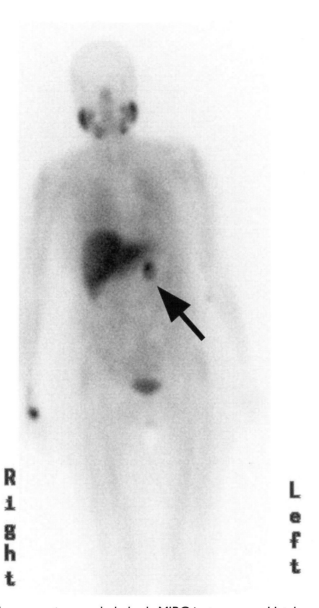

R
i
g
h
t

L
e
f
t

Phaeochromocytoma whole-body MIBG isotope scan. Uptake seen within a left adrenal phaeochromocytoma (arrow).
Note physiological uptake in the liver and salivary glands, and excretion in the bladder. The uptake over the right wrist corresponds to the injection site.

Radiological Features

- **AXR:** not generally helpful but may demonstrate a discrete, lucent, fatty mass or calcification caused by previous haemorrhage.
- **USS:** heterogeneous mass is a mix of fat and haematopoietic tissue.
- **CT:** discrete fat interspersed with fine bands of soft tissue.
- **MRI:** discrete fat is demonstrated by high signal in T1W that is suppressed on fat-suppressed sequences.

Adrenal haemorrhage

- May be caused by trauma, physiological stress (such as sepsis), a bleeding diathesis or haemorrhage into an underlying neoplasia.

Radiological features

- **USS:**
  - Especially sensitive in neonates.
  - Initially a solid mass that becomes heterogeneous through liquefaction. No signal on Doppler interrogation.
  - Chronically may have cystic appearance with echogenic calcific foci.
- **CT:**
  - Oval mass with peri-adrenal fat stranding.
  - Chronically, cystic change and calcification can occur.
- **MRI:** signal will depend on the age of haematoma and the associated blood breakdown products.

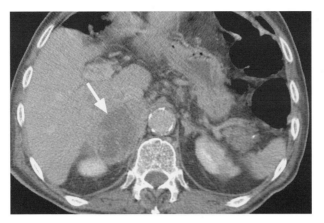

Adrenal carcinoma. Large heterogeneous right adrenal mass (arrow). The central low attenuation is secondary to necrosis.

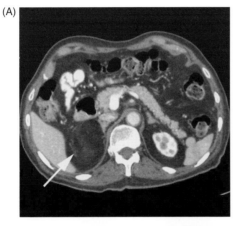

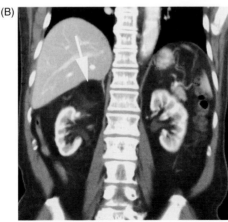

Right myelolipoma. Axial (A) and coronal (B) reformatted CECT: a large fatty mass replacing the right adrenal gland (arrows).

Aortic aneurysm

Clinical characteristics

- A focal widening of the abdominal aorta of > 3 cm, involving all layers of the vessel wall.
- Usual caused by atherosclerosis but may be secondary to trauma, infection, vasculitis or connective tissue disorders.
- Often asymptomatic.
- May present with a pulsitile mass, vessel rupture or an embolic event.
- Rupture classically presents with hypovolaemic shock, a pulsatile mass and back pain.

Radiological features

- **AXR:**
  - Calcification of the aortic wall is a common finding in atherosclerosis.
  - Loss of parallelism of the aortic wall suggests aneurysmal dilatation.
  - Rarely vertebral body erosions may be seen with long-standing aneurysms.
  - In the acute scenario, loss of the psoas outline is associated with retroperitoneal rupture.
- **USS:**
  - Is useful in both diagnosis and monitoring the size of abdominal aortic aneurysms (AAA).
  - In the acute abdomen, US can confirm the presence of an AAA, and the presence of free abdominal fluid suggests rupture.
  - However as CT is more sensitive and specific, US is most useful in the case of a patient too unstable to be transferred to CT.
- **CECT:**
  - CT is used as part of elective surgical planning in determining the anatomy of the AAA, particularly in relation to visceral vessels such as the renal arteries.
  - Retroperitoneal fibrosis associated with an AAA may be seen as a surrounding soft tissue mass.
  - In the acute setting, CT is the investigation of choice, often demonstrating the precise site of rupture and is very sensitive to intraperitoneal and retroperitoneal haemorrhage.
  - Rarer complications such as aorto-caval or aorto-enteric fistulae, and occlusion, can be detected.

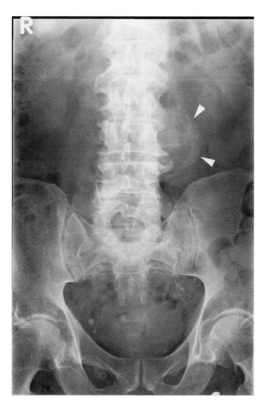

Aortic aneurysm. Calcification in the left lateral wall of the aneurysm (arrowheads).

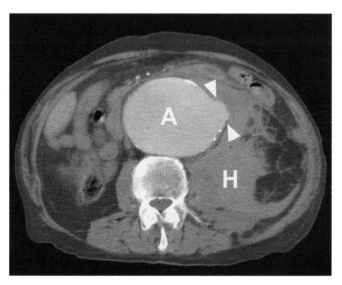

Ruptured aortic aneurysm. The arrowheads denote the breach in the wall of the aneurysm (A), with extensive associated retroperitoneal haemorrhage (H).

Appendicitis

Clinical characteristics

- A common cause of an acute abdomen with a peak incidence in the 2nd and 3rd decades.
- The aetiology is probably related to luminal obstruction, often by lymphoid hyperplasia or a faecolith.
- Typically presents with RIF pain, nausea, vomiting, fever and evidence of inflammation such as raised WBC and CRP.
- However, one-third may have an atypical presentation.
- Complications include localised perforation, abscess formation and generalised peritonitis. Rarely an obstructed appendix becomes distended by abnormal accumulation of mucus, forming an appendix mucocoele.

Radiological features

- **AXR:**
  - Is neither sensitive nor specific but can provide clues.
  - The presence of a calcified appendicolith in the RLQ, combined with abdominal pain, has a high positive predictive value for acute appendicitis.
  - Other signs are less specific and include caecal wall thickening, small-bowel ileus and decreased small-bowel gas in the RIF.
  - Free peritoneal fluid can lead to loss of the psoas outline, loss of the fat planes around the bladder and loss of definition of the inferior liver outline.

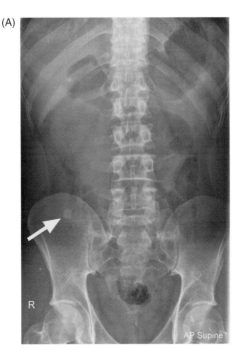

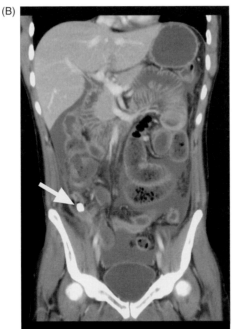

Appendicolith. AXR (A) and coronal CT reformat (B) demonstrate the presence of a RIF appendicolith (arrows). The CT demonstrates free fluid within abdomen and pelvis and several dilated loops of small bowel, secondary to ruptured appendicitis with an associated ileus.

- **USS:**
  - Is the initial imaging of choice if there is diagnostic uncertainty.
  - Can identify other causes of RIF pain such as ovarian torsion and mesenteric adenitis.
  - US findings that suggest appendicitis include:
    - visualisation of a blind-ending, non-peristaltic, non-compressible appendix.
    - a diameter of ≥6mm.
    - presence of an appendicolith, and distension of lumen.
    - peri-appendiceal free fluid.
  - **NB** A negative US does not exclude appendicitis; if there is a high degree of clinical suspicion this should not preclude further imaging or laparoscopy.

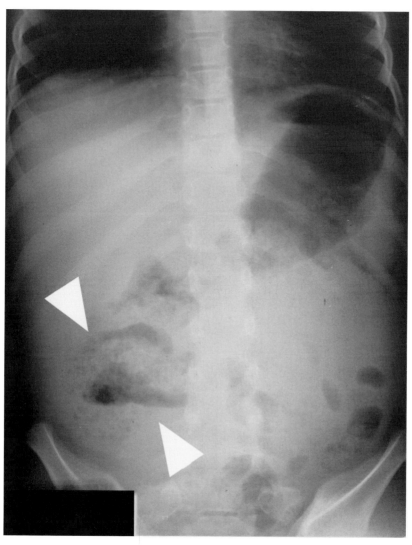

Ruptured appendicitis (arrowheads). Note the presence of an
ill-defined mottled gas pattern within the RIF, with an air–fluid level,
caused by the ruptured appendix.

- **CECT:**
  - Is increasingly being used. However, it is not a first line investigation owing to the radiation dose incurred by the patient.
  - Tends to be used where there is diagnostic dilemma such as with an atypical presentation.
  - Findings include:
    - a thickened appendix ± an appendicolith.
    - inflammatory stranding in the adjacent fat.
    - an inflammatory appendix mass.
    - a local collection.
    - local lymphadenopathy.

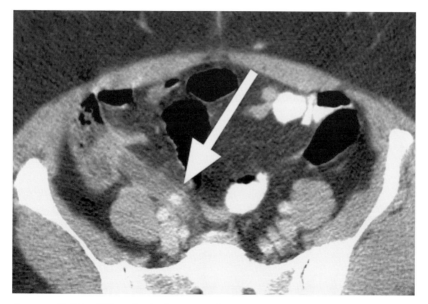

Appendicitis. Dilated tubular appendix containing an appendicolith (arrow).

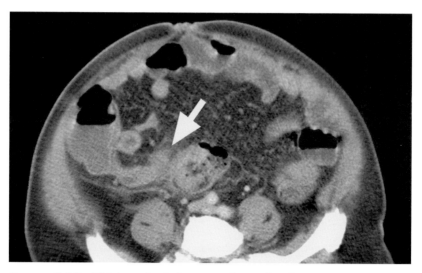

Appendicitis. Thickened tubular appendix, with inflammatory stranding seen at its tip (arrow).

Ascites

Clinical characteristics

Intra-abdominal free fluid that may be classified as:

- Exudate: >30g/dl of protein; causes include peritoneal TB, pancreatitis, Meig's syndrome and carcinomatosis.
- Transudate: <30g/dl of protein; causes include hypoalbuminaemia, congestive cardiac failure, chronic renal failure, Budd–Chiari syndrome and cirrhosis.

Radiological features

- **AXR:**
  - Initial signs relate to the dependent accumulation of free fluid in the pelvis and may be subtle and overlooked.
  - Later signs are medial displacement of both the lateral border of the liver and ascending and descending colon, bulging flanks, centralised bowel loops and a generalised 'greying' of the abdominal film.

- **USS:**
  - This is the investigation of choice to confirm the presence of ascites, without the use of ionising radiation.
  - US may provide additional information about the ascites such as loculation or the presence of debris within the fluid.
  - In addition, US allows the siting of diagnostic taps or therapeutic drains.
  - Evidence as to the aetiology of the ascites can also be gained, such as the presence of cirrhosis.

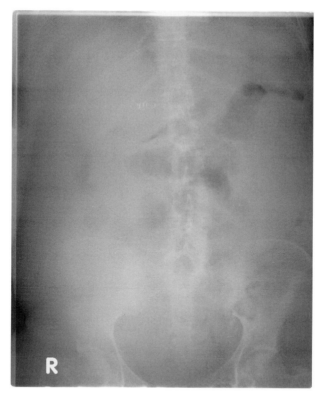

Ascites. Generalised 'greying' of the abdominal film in AXR with several centralised bowel loops.

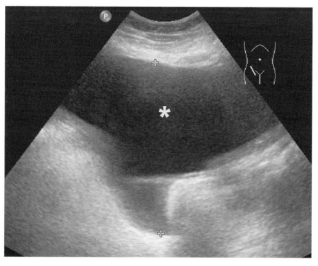

Ascites: Abdominal US showing large-volume ascites (asterisk).

- **CT:**
  - The radiation dose precludes this as an investigation to confirm the presence of ascites, but CT often confirms the presence and extent of ascites when performed for another reason.
  - The cause may also be identified, such as evidence of pancreatitis.
  - It is less sensitive than US in assessing for loculation or debris within the ascitic fluid.

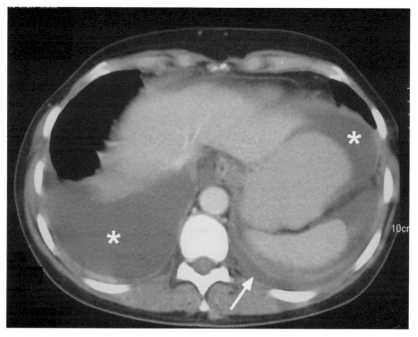

Ascites. Large-volume ascites (asterisk) and a small left basal pleural effusion in CT image (arrow).

Bezoar

Clinical characteristics

- This is an intestinal mass caused by the accumulation of ingested material.
- A phytobezoar is formed from poorly digested plant fibre.
- A trichobezoar is formed from ingested hair, almost always in females.
- Can lead to obstruction or ulceration.

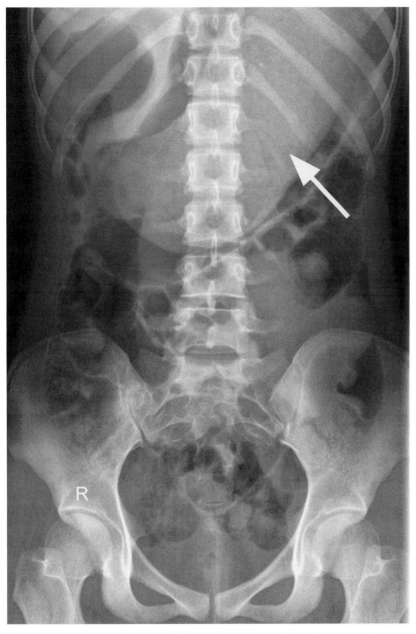

Trichobezoar. Large 'hair ball' mass completely filling the stomach (arrow).

Radiological features

- **AXR:**
  - A mass may be seen within the stomach.
  - May demonstrate bowel obstruction.
- **Barium studies:**
  - May demonstrate an intraluminal filling defect that does not have a fixed site of attachment to the bowel wall.
  - Barium may flow into crevices within the bezoar.
- **CT:**
  - This may demonstrate a low-density mass containing pockets of air.
  - As on barium studies, oral contrast may intersperse with the mass though gaps between the ingested materials.

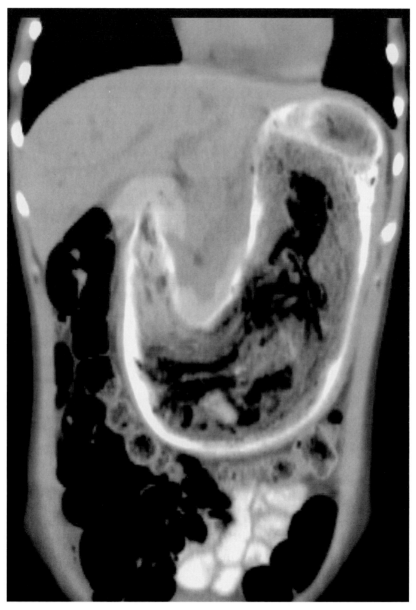

Trichobezoar (same patient) in coronal CT reformat. Oral
contrast is seen outlining the huge trichobezoar.

Biliary gas

Clinical characteristics

- Gas within the biliary tree is often an incidental finding secondary to medical intervention, such as a sphincterotomy or cholecystoenterostomy.
- Other causes include:
  - a lax sphincter of Oddi in the elderly.
  - passage of a gallstone.
  - biliary fistulae caused by stones, neoplasia or duodenal ulceration.
- Biliary gas may result in gas within the gallbladder.
- Gas within the gallbladder may be secondary to emphysematous cholecystitis. This is an infection with gas-forming organisms, seen in diabetics and leading to mural and intraluminal gallbladder gas.

Radiological features

- **AXR:** branching radiolucencies are seen within the liver. These radiolucencies do not extend to the liver edge: a feature that helps to differentiate biliary gas from gas in the portal vein. Gas in the gallbladder may result in a gas–fluid level on an erect film.
- **USS:** linear echogenic shadows, paralleling the portal venous system, are the characteristic appearance of biliary gas. Biliary calculi may be identified.
- **CT:** branching air densities that parallel the portal system will be seen. Calculi, fistulae or neoplastic masses may be identified.

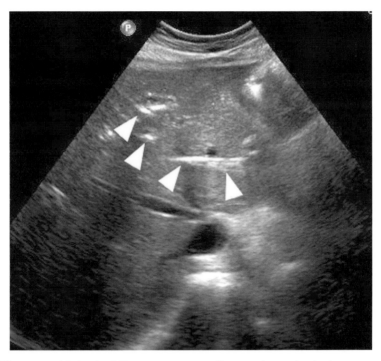

Biliary gas Air in the biliary tree seen as linear echogenic shadows paralleling the portal venous system (arrowheads).

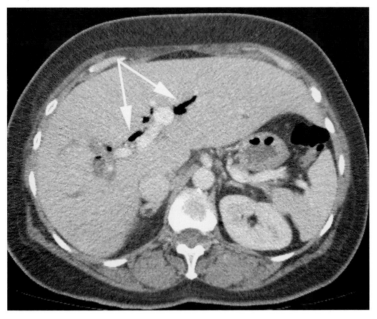

Air in the biliary tree. CT elegantly demonstrates the air (arrows). The relationship to the portal venous system is clear.

Biliary obstruction

Clinical characteristics

- Characterised by jaundice with a raised alkaline phosphatase and γ-glutamyl transferase.
- May be an acute or chronic presentation and may or may not be accompanied by pain.
- In 75% of adult biliary obstruction, the cause is benign, including calculi, strictures from previous trauma or surgery, pancreatitis and sclerosing cholangitis.
- Malignant causes include pancreatic head carcinoma, ampullary and duodenal malignancy, cholangiocarcinoma and metastases.
  - The triad of a palpable, distended gallbladder, obstructive jaundice and the absence of pain are highly suggestive of a malignant cause.
- An obstructed, infected biliary tree is a medical emergency and occurs more frequently with calculus than malignant obstruction (2:1).

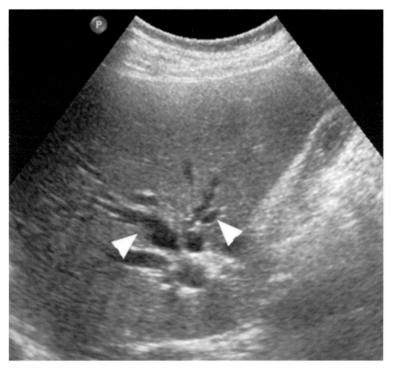

Biliary obstruction. Abdominal US demonstrating dilated biliary radicles (arrowheads) at the liver hilum.

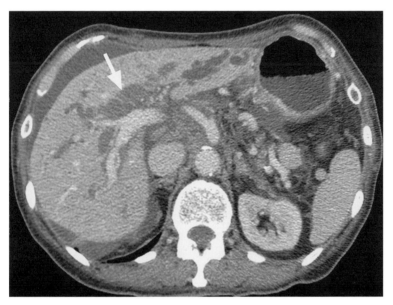

Dilatation of the biliary tree. Note the fluid-filled ducts paralleling the portal venous system (arrow).

Radiological features

- **USS:**
  - Is the imaging modality of choice in establishing the mechanical cause of biliary obstruction. The bile duct is usually easily visualised at the hepatic hilum. Most normal ducts measure <5mm in diameter; however, studies have shown that up to 4% of normal cases have a duct that measures >7mm. Therefore a diameter of 6–8mm can be non-specific and may require further investigation. Intrahepatic biliary dilatation can be seen as dilated biliary radicals seen running along the portal vessels.
  - Will often establish the cause and level of biliary obstruction, with visualisation of intraductal calculi or obstructing masses. Patient factors (such as body mass index) or overlying bowel gas may obscure the more distal biliary tree.

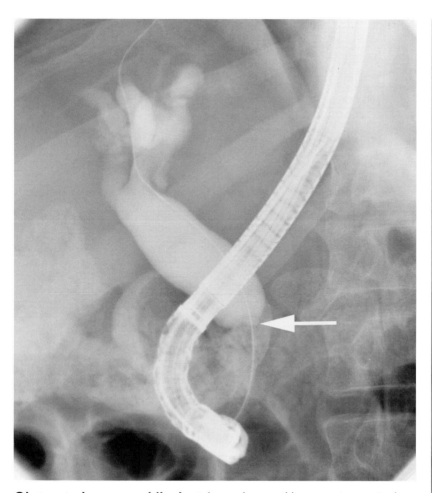

Obstructed common bile duct (arrow) caused by a carcinoma in the head of pancreas demonstrated by ERCP.

- **CT:** is sensitive for biliary tree dilatation and, although less sensitive for calculi than US, has the advantage of visualising the distal biliary tree when it is obscured on US. It can also detect, and often accurately stage, obstructing tumours.
- **Magnetic resonance cholangiopancreatography (MRCP):** use of very heavily T2W imaging sequences to outline the fluid-filled bile ducts can demonstrate the level of biliary obstruction very well. Stones are demonstrated as filling defects. The addition of conventional axial T1W and T2W images can give further information regarding extrinsic causes of obstruction such as tumours.

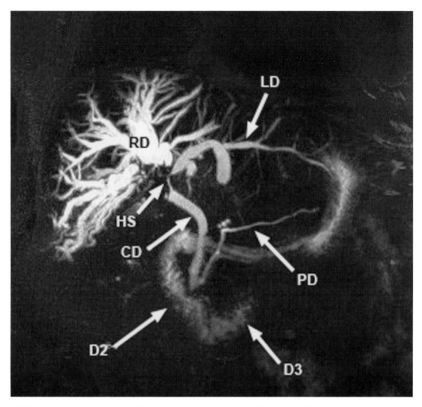

Biliary obstruction. Tight hilar stricture (HS) caused by a cholangiocarcinoma, resulting in dilatation of the right intrahepatic ducts (RD) seen by MRCP. The left intrahepatic ducts (LD) are normal by comparison but note that the tumour does cause tapering of the duct at the hilum.

CD, common duct; PD, pancreatic duct. D2 and D3, second and third parts of duodenum, respectively.

- **Endoscopic retrograde cholangiopancreatography (ERCP):** a combined endoscopic/fluoroscopic procedure outlines the biliary tree with similar effect to an MRCP, but it has the advantage of allowing therapeutic procedures such as sphincterotomy with stone removal and biliary stent placement.
- **Percutaneous trans–hepatic cholangiography (PTC):** the rise of less-invasive techniques means that PTC is now performed less as a diagnostic procedure. It is useful in patients who have had a failed ERCP and in those who cannot have an MRCP. The use of PTC has been extended to allow percutaneous trans-hepatic placement of drainage catheters or stents, especially when this is not possible during ERCP or in cases of an obstructed, infected system.

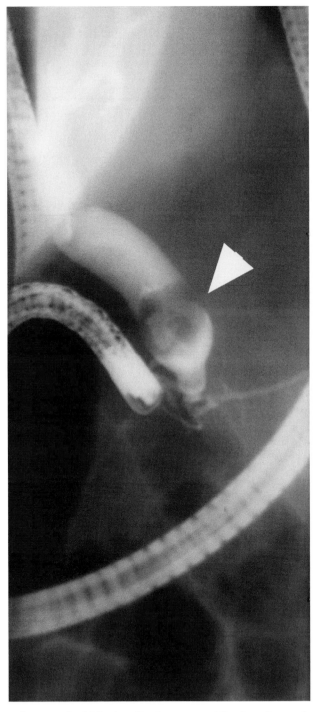

Gallstone impacted within the distal common bile duct (arrowhead) on ERCP.

Bladder calculi

Clinical characteristics

- Bladder calculi may form around a foreign body such as prostatic chippings, pubic hair, fragments of bone from penetrating injuries, and pieces of Foley catheters.
- May migrate from the proximal urinary tract.
- May be caused by stasis such as outflow obstruction, neuropathic bladders and vesicular diverticulae.
- Infection, especially with *Proteus* sp., can result in bladder calculi formation.

Radiological features

- **AXR:** Seen as a calcified body projected over the bladder area. In women, calcified fibroids may cause confusion although the latter may be seen lying above, rather than over, the bladder area.
- **USS:** Confirms the position and nature of the calcified density.

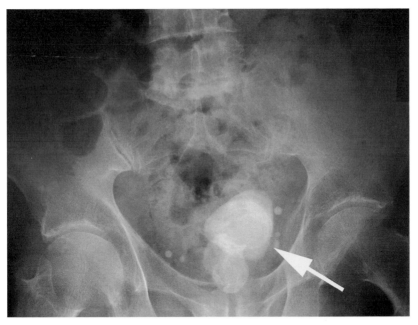

Large bilobed bladder calculus (arrow).

Bowel obstruction

Although small- and large-bowel obstruction (SBO and LBO) have common clinical features of colicky abdominal pain, vomiting, absolute constipation and abdominal distension, their aetiology and management are quite different and, therefore, will be considered separately. Predominance of certain signs depends on the level of the obstruction.

Small-bowel obstruction

Clinical characteristics

- SBO presents with colicky abdominal pain and vomiting, which occurs earlier in more proximal obstruction and later in distal obstruction.
- The bowel distal to the obstruction empties by absorption or evacuation of its contents, whereas the bowel proximal to the obstruction distends with gas and fluid.
- This eventually results in fluid shifts into the bowel, causing hypovolaemia and electrolyte imbalances.
- If SBO is not reversed it may progress from a simple to strangulated obstruction with compromise of bowel wall arterial supply with a risk of perforation and peritonitis.
- The causes of SBO can be divided into intraluminal, luminal and extrinsic causes:
  - *Intraluminal*: foreign body, bezoar, parasites, gallstones, food bolus.
  - *Luminal*: atresia, inflammatory stricture (Crohn's disease, TB), haematoma, tumour.
  - *Extrinsic*: adhesions, congenital bands, malrotation, herniae, intussusception.
- Adhesions, herniae and tumours cause the majority of SBO, with postsurgical adhesions being the most common cause.

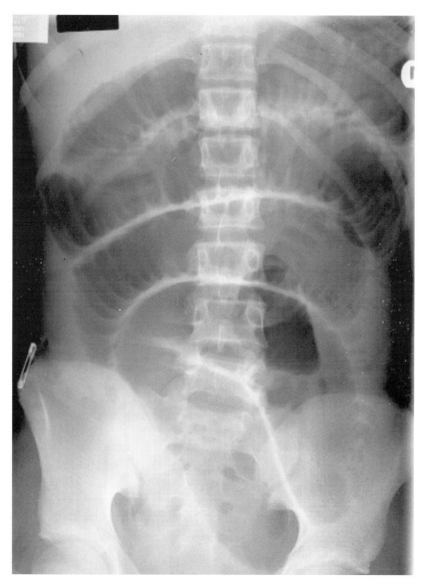

Acute small-bowel obstruction. Multiple dilated loops of small bowel within the central abdomen.

Radiological features

- **AXR:**
  - The jejunum lies mainly in the left hypochondrium and the ileum in the pelvic midline.
  - In complete SBO, the small-bowel loops will distend in 3 to 5h and are usually seen in the central abdomen.
  - An intraluminal width of >3cm on the AXR is abnormal.
  - Distended loops containing mainly fluid will appear as soft tissue density. Occasionally, small pockets of gas trapped within the valvulae conniventes create a 'string of beads' appearance.
  - A less frequent occurrence is gallstone ileus, when an intraluminal calcified stone is seen, usually in the terminal ileum, with proximal SBO and gas in the biliary tree owing to a cholecysto-duodenal fistula.
  - A closed-loop obstruction occurs when a loop of bowel is not decompressed by the caudal passage of gas and fluid. This usually occurs from adhesions and can result in a U-shaped distended loop of small bowel that does not move over time. If it contains fluid, it produces a pseudotumour appearance on the AXR because of its soft tissue density; if it contains gas, it has a coffee-bean shape.
  - In children with an intussusception, a soft tissue mass may be seen on the AXR and there may be signs of proximal SBO.
  - Chronic SBO may result in massively dilated bowel loops.
  - Intramural gas, as a result of bowel wall ischaemia, is usually associated with a poor prognosis.
  - Usually a supine AXR is sufficient for assessment of a patient with suspected SBO, but if it is normal, and there is a strong clinical suspicion of obstruction, an erect AXR may help by demonstrating air–fluid levels in dilated loops of small bowel.
  - A lateral decubitus AXR is indicated to show free gas if an erect CXR cannot be performed.

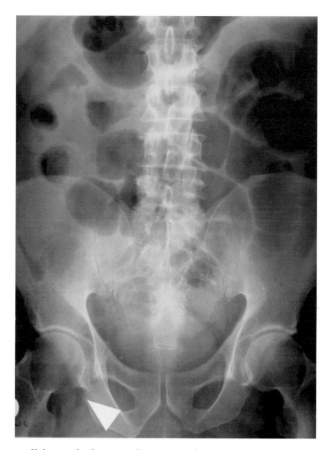

Acute small-bowel obstruction secondary to an obstructed right inguinal hernia (arrowhead).

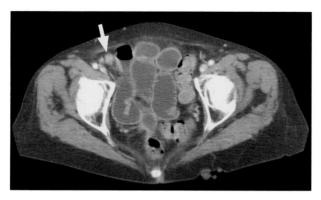

Small-bowel obstruction secondary to a right femoral hernia. The transition point is in the right femoral canal (arrow) with multiple dilated proximal loops.

- **Small bowel enema (enteroclysis):**
  - This investigation is more appropriate for chronic SBO than acute SBO and involves the placement of a nasojejunal tube and subsequent instillation of a barium suspension.
  - It will demonstrate a delay in the passage of barium and calibre change at the site of obstruction.
- **USS:**
  - Distended fluid-filled loops of small bowel are clearly visible on US and their peristaltic activity can be assessed.
  - The distal bowel loses its muscular activity at the site of obstruction, whereas proximally there is an initial increased peristalsis in an attempt to overcome the obstruction. This distinguishes it from ileus, where there is a generalised loss of peristalsis.
- **CT:**
  - When the AXR suggests SBO, CT can confirm the diagnosis, indicate the level and may reveal a cause.
  - IV contrast is given but oral contrast is not usually necessary as the dilated loops contain fluid and gas, which act as intrinsic contrast.
  - A small bowel diameter >2.5 cm on CT is abnormal.
  - A transition point, where the calibre of the bowel changes from dilated to collapsed, indicates the level of obstruction.
  - Adhesive bands are not visible on CT and the diagnosis is inferred on the basis of a transition point and the lack of an identifiable cause.
  - In closed-loop obstruction, CT will demonstrate a U-shaped loop of bowel with a slightly twisted mesentery containing vessels.
  - CT is also useful in assessing the presence of strangulation. The bowel wall will appear thickened, with oedema and haemorrhage in the mesentery. The use of IV contrast helps to assess bowel wall enhancement, and in severe cases intramural gas will be present.

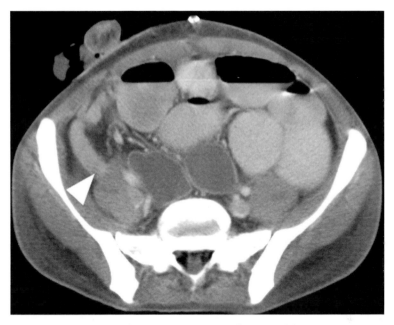

Small-bowel obstruction secondary to adhesions. Note the transition point (arrowhead) in the RIF, with multiple dilated and fluid-filled proximal small-bowel loops.

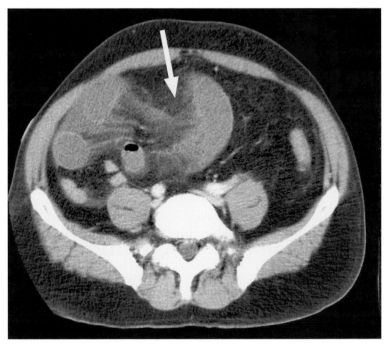

Small-bowel obstruction. Dilated fluid-filled small-bowel loops secondary to a closed loop obstruction (arrow).

Large bowel obstruction

Clinical characteristics

- Abdominal distension predominates, with colicky abdominal pain, and absolute constipation a feature of complete obstruction.
- Faeculent vomiting occurs if the ileocaecal valve is incompetent, when the features of SBO are added to those of LBO.
- The most common causes of LBO are carcinoma of the colon, diverticulitis and volvulus, with carcinoma being the most common.
- The clinical history may suggest the underlying cause: an abrupt onset of symptoms suggests an acute event such as volvulus, a history of change in bowel habit and weight loss suggests carcinoma, and a chronic history of constipation suggests diverticulitis.
- Right-sided colonic lesions can become quite large before obstruction develops owing to the soft stool consistency, whereas sigmoid and rectal tumours obstruct earlier because of the narrower colonic calibre and more solid stool.

Radiological features

- **AXR:**
  - This may be diagnostic. The distended colon lies around the periphery of the abdomen and is distinguished from small bowel by haustral markings that do not traverse the entire bowel lumen.
  - Bowel distal to the obstruction is collapsed and the rectum does not contain gas.
  - If there is a tumour of the caecum and ascending colon, with an incompetent ileocaecal valve, only the small bowel may be distended.
  - The typical appearance of a caecal or sigmoid volvulus may be apparent (this is covered elsewhere).
  - Intramural or free intra-abdominal gas may be seen.
- **Water-soluble contrast enema:**
  - A water-soluble contrast rather than barium is used because of the risk of intraperitoneal contamination when perforation has occurred; the contrast is instilled rectally.
  - It may confirm the diagnosis and indicate the level of obstruction.
  - In most instances, contrast enemas have been replaced by abdominal and pelvic CT studies.

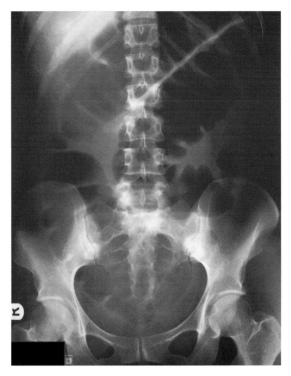

Large-bowel obstruction. Gaseous distension of the colon, with relative paucity of air beyond the mid descending colon.

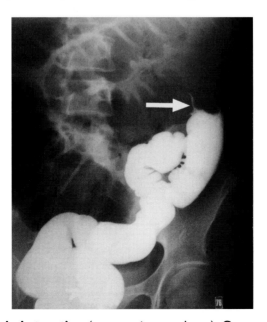

Large-bowel obstruction (same patient as above). Contrast enema demonstrates an obstructing lesion (arrow) within the mid descending colon.

- **USS:** may demonstrate fluid-filled loops of bowel and thickened bowel wall, but the findings are often non-specific and generally not helpful.
- **CT:**
  - This has advantages over contrast enema especially in elderly or frail patients.
  - It is usually performed with IV contrast; oral contrast may be helpful to outline small-bowel loops.
  - CT will confirm the obstruction, with a colonic diameter of >6cm (9cm in the caecum) being considered abnormal.
  - The identification of a transition point indicates the level and the cause may also be apparent.
  - As stated above, the most common cause is colonic carcinoma, followed by diverticulitis and volvulus.
  - One of the limitations of CT is the difficulty in differentiating diverticulitis from colonic cancer in certain patients.
  - CT will also assess the presence of complications, such as strangulation, as indicated by congestive changes or haemorrhage in the mesentery, bowel wall thickening, and intramural gas.

Pseudo-obstruction

Clinical characteristics

- Also known as Ogilvie syndrome, this is a clinical syndrome with the signs, symptoms and radiographic appearance of LBO but with no identifiable mechanical cause.
- Recognised causes are:
  - recent surgery.
  - severe pulmonary or cardiovascular disease.
  - severe electrolyte disturbance: hyponatraemia, hypokalaemia, hypomagnesaemia, hypo/hypercalcaemia.
  - malignancy.
  - systemic infection.
  - severe constipation.
  - medications: opioids, anticholinergic drugs, clonidine, amphetamines, phenothiazines, steroids.

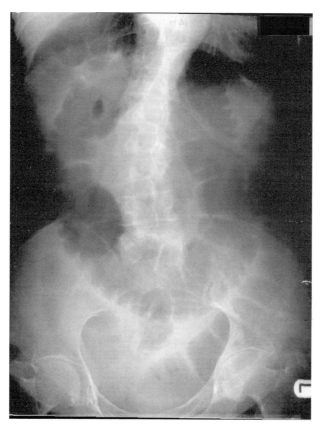

Large-bowel obstruction secondary to an obstructing sigmoid carcinoma. Note the extensive colonic distension up to, and including, the sigmoid colon.

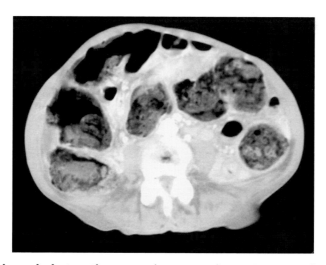

Large-bowel obstruction secondary to an obstructing sigmoid carcinoma, with extensive colonic dilatation and gross faecal loading.

Radiological features

- **AXR:**
  - This does not differentiate pseudo-obstruction from mechanical obstruction but will demonstrate distended loops of large bowel.
  - Serial films may be useful to document the clinical course and monitor the colonic diameter.
- **Water-soluble contrast enema:** a water-soluble contrast enema will not only help to exclude a mechanical obstruction, by demonstrating free passage of contrast, but may also be therapeutic when Gastrografin is used, as its hyperosmolality causes a fluid shift into the bowel, stimulating colonic motility.
- **CT:** further imaging is not usually necessary unless a mechanical obstruction has not yet been excluded.

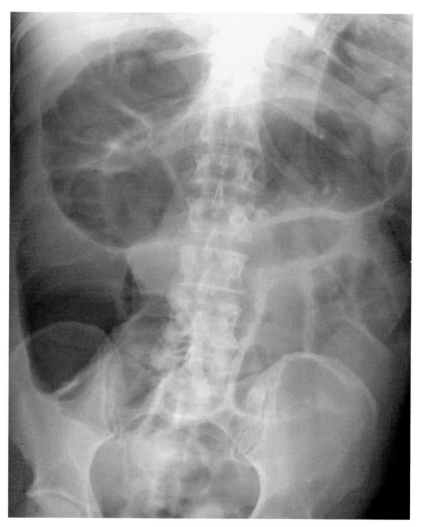

Pseudo-obstruction. Significant gaseous distension of the ascending and transverse colon. In contrast with mechanical large-bowel obstruction, no obstructing lesion can be identified to account for the appearances.

Ileus

Clinical characteristics

- Paralytic ileus usually occurs after intra–abdominal surgery but may also occur in several other settings:
  - Postoperative: most common.
  - Inflammatory bowel disease.
  - Inflammatory: pancreatitis, appendicitis, cholecystitis, diverticulitis, peritonitis.
  - Metabolic: hypokalaemia, hypocalcaemia, hypomagnesaemia.
  - Medication: opioids.
- It occurs due to cessation of peristalsis, resulting in a functional obstruction.
- It differs from pseudo-obstruction in that both the small and large bowel are involved.
- The patient presents with abdominal distension and vomiting, usually postoperatively.
- Colicky pain is not a feature and bowel sounds are absent, in contrast to the high-pitched sounds of obstruction.

Radiological features

- **AXR:**
  - Loops of both small and large bowel will be dilated with no apparent transition point.
  - Further imaging is only necessary if there is difficulty excluding a mechanical obstruction.

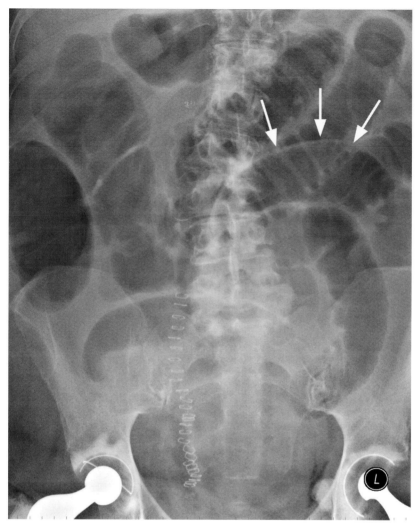

Ileus. Postoperative gaseous distension of both small and large bowel. Note the midline surgical staples and the positive Rigler's sign (arrows).

Calcifications

Numerous structures can calcify within the abdomen and pelvis. Most of these are of no importance, but raise clinical concern when the AXR is viewed!

- **Costochondral calcification:** age–related calcification of the costo-chondral junctions is a common finding in the lower ribs projecting over the superior part of the AXR. Typically in men, the calcification is parallel to the edge of the cartilage, while in women the calcification is central.
- **Fibroid calcification:** degenerate uterine fibroids (leiomyomata) may calcify, resulting in a rounded, lobulated calcific body projected over the female pelvis.
- **Haematoma:** some haematomas heal leaving a residual area of calci-fication. Haematomas that follow an intramuscular injection into the buttocks often calcify and may project over the pelvis and lower abdo-men, possibly leading to diagnostic concern. These haematomas are usually well defined, rounded or oval with rim calcification.

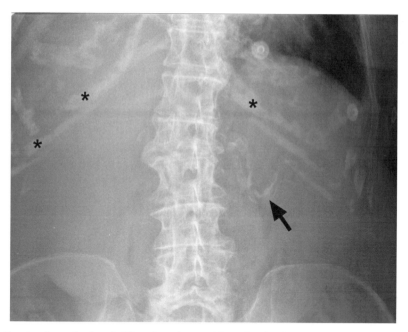

Costochondral calcification (asterisk) and **splenic artery** (arrow) **calcification**.

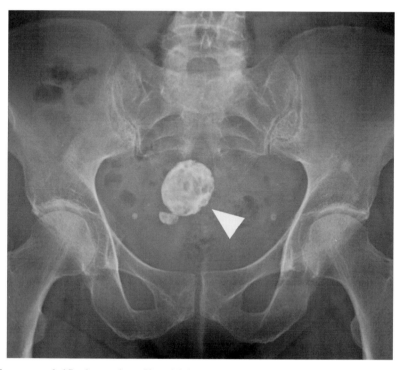

Large calcified uterine fibroid (arrowhead).

- **Mesenteric lymph nodes:** postinflammatory nodes may calcify. If mesenteric nodes are affected this may result in lobulated calcification, which typically lies medially within the abdomen. This may cause diagnostic confusion particularly in gallstone ileus. Calcified mesenteric nodes are not evidence of active lymph node disease.
- **Phleboliths:** phleboliths are benign venous calcifications that commonly occur in the pelvic veins and may simulate distal ureteric stones. A typical phlebolith is round with a slightly radiolucent centre. However, they may be projected over the course of the lower ureter and those with an atypical appearance may be indistinguishable from ureteric stones. If this is a clinical concern, further imaging, such as an IVU or non-enhanced CT, may be necessary.

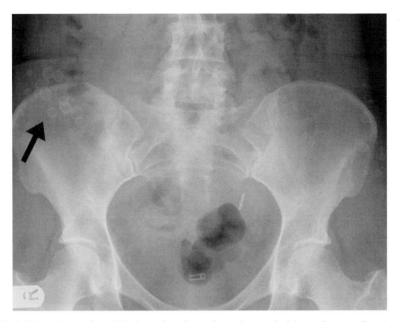

Calcification of multiple injection sites (arrow). Note the sterilisation clips within the pelvis.

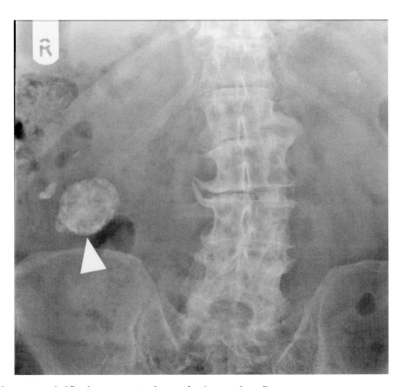

Large calcified mesenteric node (arrowhead).

- **Transverse processes:** clearly calcification is normal in the transverse processes of the lumbar vertebrae. However, the tips often appear denser on AXR than the remainder of the transverse processes and can, on occasion, be misinterpreted as ureteric calculi, as the courses of the ureters often overlie the lower four transverse processes.
- **Vascular calcification:** vascular calcification is a common finding, particularly in the elderly. Typically is seen as parallel lines of calcification running along the course of arterial structures, most commonly the aorta and iliac arteries. Often in the elderly these vessels have an ectatic course, but the parallel nature of the calcification remains. If parallelism is lost, aneurysmal dilatation should be suspected. The splenic artery is often seen as a calcified serpiginous vessel in the left upper quadrant.

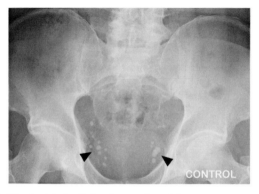

Multiple calcified phleboliths (arrowheads).

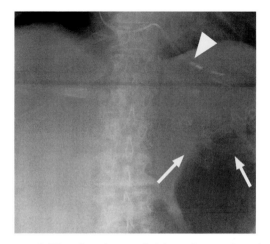

Splenic artery calcification (arrows). Note the incidental pacemaker lead (arrowhead).

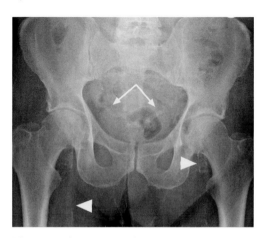

Vascular calcification (arrowheads) and **seminal vesical** (arrows) calcification.

Chilaiditi's sign/syndrome

Clinical characteristics

- Pronounced 'Ky-la-ditty'.
- Refers to the usually asymptomatic interposition of bowel between the liver and right hemidiaphragm; usually is hepatic flexure, less commonly small bowel.
- Seen in up to 0.25% of chest CXRs.
- Most frequently an incidental finding in males and almost always in adults.
- Contributing factors include:
  - absence of normal suspensory ligaments of the transverse colon.
  - abnormality or absence of the falciform ligament.
  - redundant colon, as might be seen in chronic constipation.
  - aerophagia (air 'swallower').
  - paralysis or eventration of the right hemidiaphragm.
  - chronic lung disease, cirrhosis and ascites.
- *Chilaiditi's 'sign'* refers to the asymptomatic presence of interposed bowel.
- *Chilaiditi's 'syndrome'* may present with:
  - abdominal pain.
  - constipation.
  - vomiting.
  - respiratory distress.
  - anorexia.
- It is clinically important because it may simulate a pneumoperitoneum, resulting in unnecessary surgery.

Radiological features

- **CXR:** the presence of haustral folds within the 'air beneath the diaphragm' confirms it is contained within large bowel.

- **CT:**
  - May be required if there is diagnostic dilemma.
  - Particularly useful if there is strong clinical suspicion of concomitant pneumoperitoneum, as this may be more difficult to diagnose.

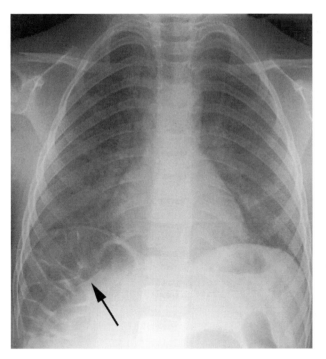

Chilaiditi's sign. CXR shows interposition of hepatic flexure between the liver and right hemidiaphragm (arrow). Note the presence of multiple colonic haustrations.

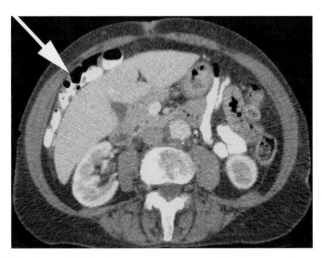

Chilaiditi's sign. CECT shows interposition of the hepatic flexure between the liver and right hemidiaphragm (arrow).

Cholecystitis

Clinical characteristics

- Inflammation of the gallbladder that presents with RUQ pain.
- May be acute or chronic; the most common aetiology is gallstones in both.
  - In acute cholecystitis, gallstones impact in the neck of gallbladder or within the cystic duct, with spontaneous disimpaction in 85%.
  - Complications include perforation, gallbladder necrosis and gallbladder empyema.
- acalculous cholecystitis may be caused by decreased flow in the cystic artery, occurs more common in seriously ill patients, can be complicated by perforation and has a 6% mortality rate.

Radiological features

- **USS:** mainstay of imaging in cholecystitis.
  - Primary finding is of a thickened gallbladder wall (>3mm), which may be poorly defined, with impacted calculi.
  - A gallstone is identified as an echogenic body with posterior acoustic shadowing.
  - The presence of inflammatory fluid or exudate surrounding the gallbladder is often seen.
  - Inflammatory debris may be identified as coarse non-dependent echogenic material that, unlike stones, has no acoustic shadow.
  - Positive ultrasound Murphy's sign in 85% Focal gallbladder tenderness upon direct pressure with the US probe.

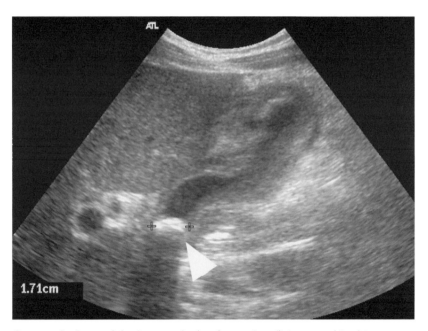

Acute cholecystitis. Large calculus (arrowhead) impacted in the neck of the gallbladder. Associated thickened and oedematous gallbladder wall.

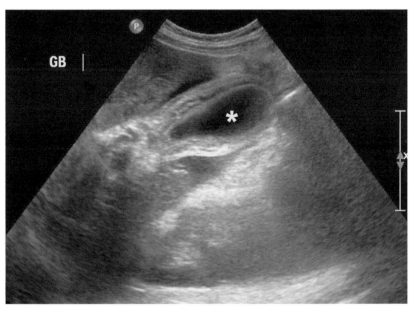

Acalculus cholecystitis (asterisk). Markedly thickened and oedematous gallbladder wall with surrounding pericholecystic free fluid.

- **CT:** should not be necessary in the investigation of cholecystitis but may be utilised as part of the investigation of non-specific abdominal pain.
  - Again the primary finding is of gallbladder mural thickening. Associated inflammatory changes may be seen, characterised by stranding in the adjacent fat. Biliary calculi may be identified.
  - CT may be used to assess for complications such as perforation or necrosis.
- **MRI:** can be helpful in difficult cases.
  - MRCP may demonstrate biliary calculi.
  - Standard MRI sequences may demonstrate gallbladder wall thickening; T2W scans, with fat suppression, can show associated inflammatory changes and pericholecystic fluid.

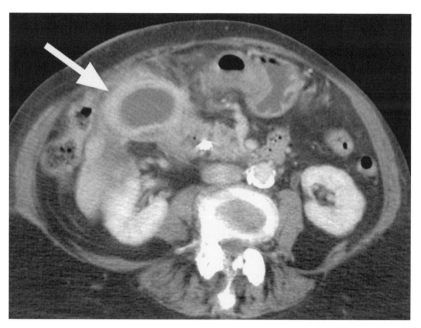

Acute cholecystitis; CT features. Markedly thickened enhancing gallbladder wall (arrow), with associated surrounding inflammatory stranding.

Cirrhosis

Clinical characteristics

- Cirrhosis is defined as hepatic fibrosis with the formation of regenerative nodules lacking normal hepatic architecture; particularly lack of a central vein.
- The aetiology is varied but a common underlying factor is repeated or chronic inflammation and tissue destruction, with subsequent disorganised repair and regeneration.
- There is a huge variety of causative agents. In developed countries, the most common are viral (hepatitis B) and toxic (chronic alcohol abuse). In some cases, no cause is found (cryptogenic hepatic cirrhosis).
- Other less-common causes include;
  - infestation with Schistosomes.
  - chronic biliary obstruction; inflammatory bowel disease, cystic fibrosis, primary biliary cirrhosis.
  - haemochromatosis.
  - vascular insufficiency from hepatic veno-occlusive disease or congestive heart failure.
  - nutritional: intestinal bypass procedures, abetalipoproteinaemia and steatosis.
  - drug-induced: particularly with methotrexate, isoniazid and methyldopa.
  - genetic: Wilson's disease, type IV glycogen storage disease and α_1-antitrypsin deficiency.
- A pseudo-cirrhotic picture is seen in patients with treated hepatic metastatic disease and should not be confused with real hepatic cirrhosis.
- Morphologically there are two main types of cirrhosis:
  - **Chronic sclerosing cirrhosis** involves minimal regeneration of hepatocytes with little nodule formation leading to a small hard liver.
  - **Nodular cirrhosis** shows significant regeneration, leading to the formation of multiple small nodules. In the early stages, the liver may be enlarged.
- Deranged intrahepatic venous flow results in bypassing of portal venous flow directly into the systemic vasculature, leading to the development of submucosal porto-venous varices, most commonly in the distal oesophagus and rectal mucosa.
- Patients present with signs and symptoms of chronic liver failure and complications from portal hypertension.
- Clinical features include jaundice, low-grade fever, anorexia and weight loss, and nephrotic syndrome caused by low serum albumin (deficient production by the liver).

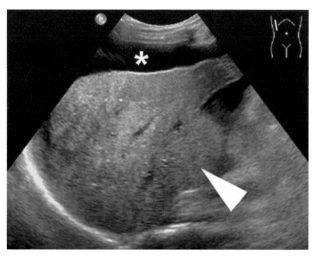

Cirrhosis. Shrunken liver with an irregular margin and coarsened echotexture. Note the presence of caudate lobe hypertrophy (arrowhead) and ascites (asterisk).

- Clinical features of portal hypertension include hepatic encephalopathy (from bypassing of the liver's detoxifying capability secondary to porto-systemic shunts) and risk of significant, often life-threatening, haemorrhage from oesophageal or rectal varices.
- There is an association with hypogonadism, anaemia, pancreatitis, coagulopathy and cholelithiasis.

Radiological features

- Radiological features include changes visible within the liver, changes owing to portal hypertension and changes from chronic hepatic insufficiency.
- **AXR:** some of these changes, such as initial hepatic enlargement, ascites and splenomegaly, may be seen on plain radiography but this is not sensitive or specific.
- **USS:**
  - US has an overall sensitivity of 80% in the detection of changes from cirrhosis.
  - On US, the liver may be enlarged initially with subsequent shrinkage noted.
  - Because of differential portal supply, the right lobe is often more affected than the left, with subsequent shrinkage of the right lobe (including the quadrate lobe), with hypertrophy of the left lobe and caudate lobe (segment 1).
  - Surface nodularity, increased parenchymal echogenicity, a coarse heterogeneous texture and surface indentations are all seen on USS.

- Coexisting splenomegaly and signs of portal hypertension such as portal varices and ascites are common.
- On duplex imaging, there is generally increased hepatic arterial resistance following a meal and so-called 'portalisation' of the hepatic venous waveform.
- **CT:**
  - On CECT, a shrunken liver with an irregular drawn-in surface is generally seen. Liver density and enhancement following IV contrast is variable.
  - Fatty infiltration as seen in early cirrhosis may lead to a hypodense enlarged liver. Generally there is non-uniform enhancement owing to areas of fatty infiltration and areas of hepatic fibrosis.
  - Hypertrophy of the caudate lobe may be seen.
  - Liver density may, however, be normal. Splenomegaly and ascites are easily detected by CECT.
- **MRI:** is often used as a problem-solving tool in liver imaging, and cirrhosis is no exception.
  - An irregular area within the liver, as seen on US and CECT, may represent a regenerating cirrhotic nodule, a dysplastic nodule or a frankly malignant nodule (cirrhosis is a strong risk factor for the development of hepatocellular carcinoma, particularly if caused by viral infection).
  - Regenerating nodules are hypointense on T1W and T2W sequences because of iron deposits within them. Malignant nodules tend to be variable on T1W and hyperintense on T2W images. They show marked early contrast enhancement following gadolinium on T1W sequences.

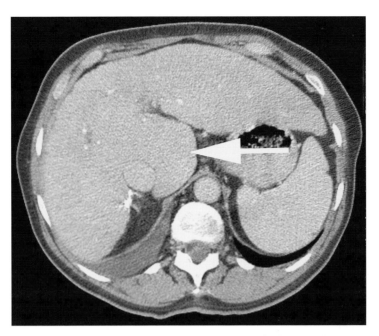

Cirrhosis. Axial scan in the portal phase. As on US, the liver has an irregular in-drawn margin and there is hypertrophy of the caudate lobe. Note that the liver is generally of reduced attenuation in comparison with the spleen, consistent with diffuse fatty infiltration.

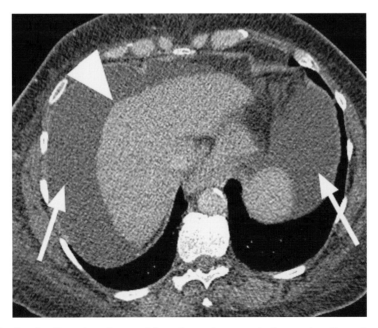

Cirrhosis. Shrunken liver, with an irregular margin (arrowhead), and ascites (arrows).

Colitis

- Colitis is inflammation of the colon.
- Causes include inflammatory bowel disease, ischaemia and infection.

Ulcerative colitis

Clinical characteristics

- Ulcerative colitis (UC) is an idiopathic inflammatory bowel disease that affects the colon and usually starts in the rectum. It causes circumferential, continuous proximal inflammation of the colon and, unlike Crohn's disease, skip lesions are not a feature.
- The diagnosis is usually made using endoscopy and biopsy.
- There may be a backwash terminal ileitis but otherwise GI involvement is limited to the colon.
- Presents with abdominal pain and bloody diarrhoea. May be accompanied by electrolyte imbalances and fevers.
- The usual pattern is of periods of disease activity interspersed with periods of remission.
- There are extra-colonic manifestations, which include erythema nodosum, iritis, primary sclerosing cholangitis, chronic active hepatitis, peripheral arthritis and spondylitis.
- Complications include toxic megacolon, with its associated high risk of perforation and death. More chronic complications include stricture formation and markedly increased risk of colonic carcinoma.

Radiological features

- **AXR:** plain films may demonstrate hyperplastic 'mucosal islands'; diffuse colonic dilatation, with loss of the normal haustral pattern; and paucity of faecal material owing to inflammation.
- **Barium enema (acute phase):** may demonstrate narrowing and incomplete filling owing to spasm. Different types of ulcer may be seen: undermining (collar stud) ulcers, shallow ulcers or longitudinal submucosal ulceration, resulting in a double tract of barium. Fine granularity of the mucosa may be seen owing to a combination of mucosal oedema and fine ulceration. Oedematous haustra may result in thumb printing. Pseudopolyps may be caused by oedematous areas of mucosa separated by areas of denuded mucosa.
- **Barium enemas (chronic stage):** may demonstrate a featureless, narrow-calibre lumen – 'hose pipe' colon. Malignant transformation may be seen. Surveillance for malignant change is usually via endoscopy, thus avoiding radiation in what is often a young population.
- **CT:** may demonstrate circumferential wall thickening >10mm. A continuous distribution from the rectum is suggestive of UC.

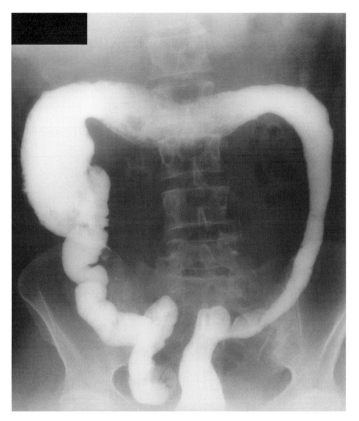

Late-stage ulcerative colitis. Single contrast enema demonstrates an extensive featureless colon with loss of haustrations, narrowing of the lumen and associated shortening. There is also mucosal irregularity in the transverse colon consistent with ulceration.

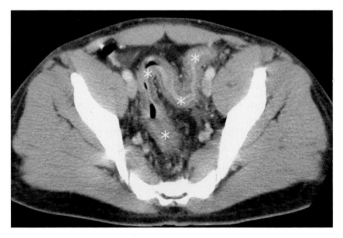

Ulcerative colitis. Diffuse circumferential colonic wall thickening (asterixes) due to UC.

Differential diagnosis

One of the main differential diagnoses for UC is Crohn's disease

Differences between UC and Crohn's disease

Feature	Crohn's disease	Ulcerative colitis
GI tract	Can affect any segment	Colon and reflux terminal ileitis only
Skip lesions	Present	None; continuous starting at distal colon
Colonic shortening	None	Yes, plus loss of haustra in chronic cases
Ulcers	Deep, fissuring	Shallow confluent
Fistulae	A feature	None
Pseudodiverticulum	Yes	None
Toxic megacolon	Rare	Relatively common
Carcinoma	Slight increase in colonic carcinoma rate	Marked increase in rate of colonic adenocarcinoma

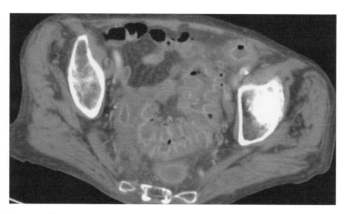

Pseudomembranous colitis. Marked circumferential sigmoid colonic wall thickening with mucosal enhancement.

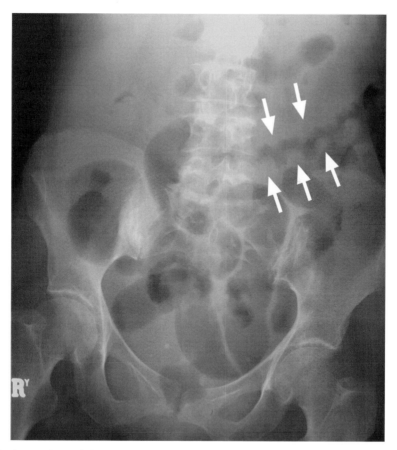

Ischaemic colitis. Note the characteristic 'thumb printing' of thickened, oedematous folds in the distal transverse colon (arrows).

Pseudomembranous colitis

Clinical characteristics

- Colitis induced by a toxin produced by *Clostridium difficile*.
- Predisposing factors include antibiotic therapy, shock, proximal LBO, intestinal ischaemia and renal transplantation.
- Results in profuse watery diarrhoea, abdominal pain and tenderness.
- Endoscopy shows pseudomembranes.
- Diagnosed by visualisation of the pseudomembranes and stool assay for the toxin.

Radiological features

- **AXR:** may demonstrate an ileus with mild gaseous large and small bowel distension. Thumb printing may be a feature. The haustra may appear thickened owing to oedema and the pseudomembranes may cause an irregular, shaggy mucosal appearance.
- **Barium enema:** generally not required and is contraindicated in severe cases. May demonstrate barium within clefts in the pseudomembranes. The pseudomembranes may cause a nodular or shaggy appearance.
- **USS:** may demonstrate non-specific colonic wall thickening and the presence of ascites.
- **CT**: may demonstrate circumferential colonic wall thickening with mucosal enhancement.

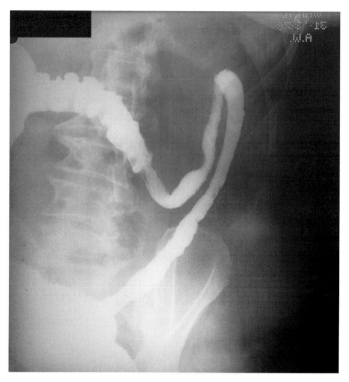

Late-stage ischaemic colitis. Single-contrast barium enema demonstrates a clear zone of transition between normal and abnormal colon at the junction of the middle and distal thirds of the transverse colon. The proximal colon has normal mucosa and haustral pattern while the distal segment is featureless and abnormally narrowed.

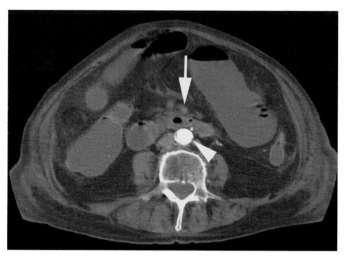

Superior mesenteric artery (SMA) thrombosis. Normal enhancement of the aorta (arrowhead). No enhancement seen in the SMA (arrow).

Ischaemic colitis

Clinical characteristics

- Ischaemic colitis is caused by interruption to the colonic blood supply.
- Aetiologies include thrombosis, bowel obstruction and trauma.
- Predisposing factors include age, oral contraceptives, sickle cell disease and surgical ligation of the inferior mesenteric artery.
- Presents with acute lower abdominal pain and tenderness, usually out of proportion to the clinical signs. There may be rectal bleeding or diarrhoea.
- Most commonly affects the left side of the colon, especially at the splenic flexure where there is a watershed between the territories of the superior and inferior mesenteric arteries. The rectum is usually spared.
- May be a transient condition with spontaneous resolution over a few months. May lead to incomplete healing with smooth stricture formation. Severe disease can lead to colonic infarction, with a high associated mortality.

Radiological features

- **AXR:** plain film is often normal; however, gas within the colon may outline the characteristic thumb printing of thickened, oedematous folds seen in this condition.
- **Barium enema:** single-contrast instant enema may demonstrate thumb printing and ulceration associated with this condition. A double-contrast enema shows these findings more reliably but should be used with caution in an acutely ill patient. A smooth stricture may be demonstrated on a delayed study.
- **CT:** contrast-enhanced spiral CT is the usual first-line investigation for suspected ischaemic colitis. A dual phase scan, performed in the arterial and portal phases, may demonstrate thrombus in both the mesenteric arterial or venous systems. The affected colon may appear abnormally circumferentially thickened and demonstrate poor contrast enhancement. There may be a sharp cut off between normal and abnormal colon at the boundary of vascular territories. Mural gas may be seen in more advanced disease and, in severe cases, portal gas may be identified. The latter is a poor prognostic factor.
- **Angiography:** a more limited role in the era of multislice spiral CT but may demonstrate attenuated arterial flow or the presence of a thrombus.

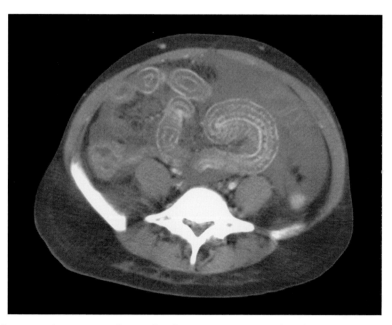

Mesenteric venous thrombosis: extensive serosal and mucosal enhancement caused by mesenteric venous thrombosis.

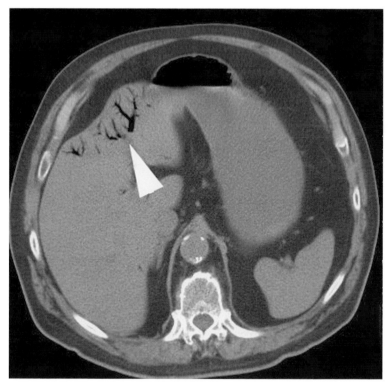

Bowel necrosis. Portal venous gas (arrowhead) secondary to necrosis.

Radiation colitis

Clinical characteristics

- A late complication of radiotherapy that may present many years after therapy. Typically involves doses of > 45 Gy.
- The radiation causes an occlusive endarteritis.
- Most commonly occurs in the rectum following treatment of gynaecological malignancy.
- May cause rectal bleeding, tenesmus and diarrhoea.

Radiological features

- Changes are confined to the radiotherapy field.
- **Barium enema:** may show strictures; these will often be smooth and symmetrical, but prior ulceration may lead to scarring and distortion of colonic folds. Fistulae may also occur.
- **CT:** may demonstrate luminal narrowing and homogeneous colonic wall thickening. There may be thickening of pararectal fascia by fibrosis. The surrounding fat may show increased density, again from fibrosis.

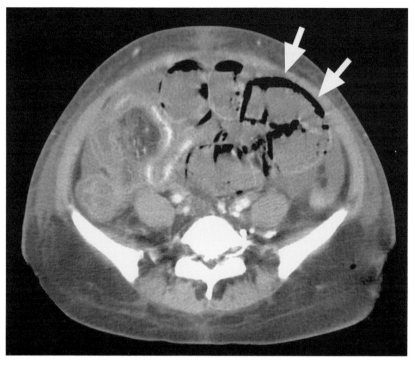

Small-bowel infarction with the development of extensive mural gas
(arrows).

Toxic megacolon

Clinical characteristics

- This is an acute fulminant full-thickness colitis.
- There is loss of smooth muscle tone, with rapid development of extensive colonic dilatation (>5.5 cm).
- Most commonly seen in UC.
- Other causes include Crohn's disease, ischaemic colitis, pseudomembranous colitis and infective colitis.
- Untreated, this results in colonic perforation, with an associated mortality of 20%.

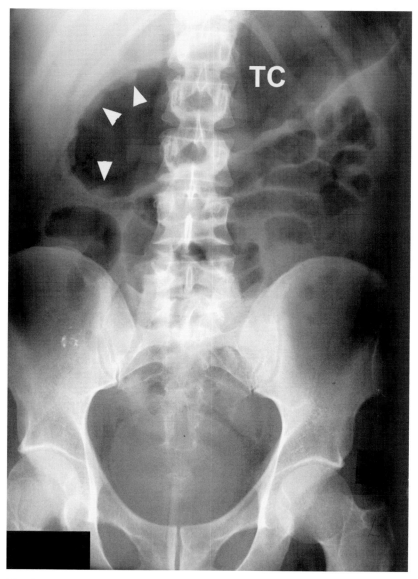

Toxic megacolon. Oedematous mucosal 'islands' (arrowheads) seen in a dilated transverse colon (TC).

Radiological features

- **AXR:** plain films demonstrate colonic distension/colonic ileus. This may be localised or involve the whole colon. The loss of the normal haustral pattern and development of mucosal islands suggests mucosal ischaemia. Mural gas and free peritoneal gas are late complications.
- **Serial AXR:** may demonstrate increasing dilatation. Associated small-bowel dilatation indicates poor prognosis for medical treatment.
- **CT:** demonstrates colonic dilatation, with distorted haustra and mucosal islands. Late complications such as mural gas and free intraperitoneal air are readily identifiable.
- **Barium enema: contraindicated** because of the risk of perforation.

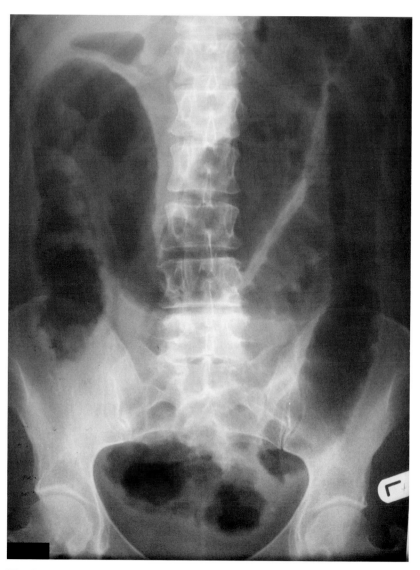

Toxic megacolon. Extensive colonic distenstion with multiple mucosal 'islands' throughout, indicating developing mucosal ischaemia; this is usually a precursor to perforation.

Colonic carcinoma

Clinical characteristics

- Most common GI carcinoma. Causes 15% of cancer deaths.
- Predisposing conditions include familial polyposis coli, Gardner's syndrome and inflammatory bowel disease.
- Presentations include weight loss, iron-deficiency anaemia, abdominal pain, rectal bleeding, perforation, intussusception and colonic obstruction.
- Common sites for secondary spread include liver, lung, lymph nodes and adrenals.

Radiological features

- **AXR:** useful in secondary large-bowel obstruction but otherwise AXR has a non-specific role in diagnosing colonic carcinoma.
- **Barium enema:** double-contrast barium enema has, in the past, been the radiological investigation of choice. May demonstrate the classic annular 'apple core' lesion or a fungating polypoid lesion. Rarely, longitudinal and circumferential spread (scirrhous carcinoma) is seen, especially related to chronic UC.

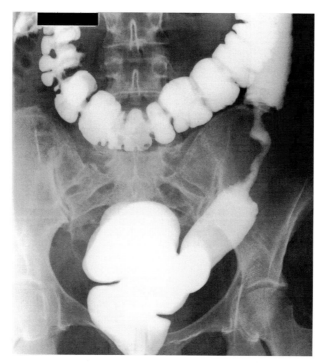

Colonic carcinoma. 'Apple core' stricture of the mid descending colon caused by a carcinoma.

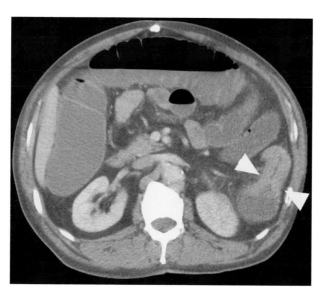

Annular carcinoma at the splenic flexure (arrowheads) resulting in proximal large-bowel obstruction; note the dilated fluid-filled proximal colon.

- **USS:** can detect large carcinomas, nodal and hepatic spread, but is relatively insensitive for primary colonic carcinoma.
- **CT pneumocolon:** excellent investigation for demonstrating the abnormal mural thickening of colonic carcinoma. It has the advantage over barium enemas of being able to demonstrate extra-colonic involvement, and incidental non-colonic pathology.
- **Standard CECT:**
  - Can demonstrate the larger carcinomas, and oral contrast 24h prior to the scan increases the sensitivity. Psammomatous calcification may be seen in mucinous adenocarcinoma.
  - Can accurately stage colonic carcinoma, including intrathoracic spread.
  - Complications such as perforation, obstruction and abscess formation can be assessed.

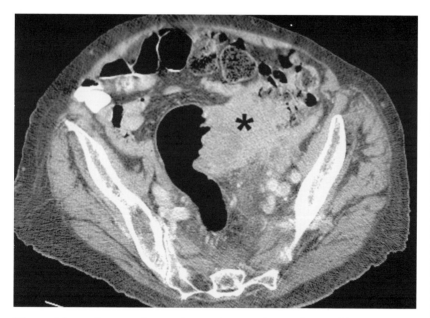

Sigmoid carcinoma. Large obstructing carcinoma (asterisk). See the following three related images.

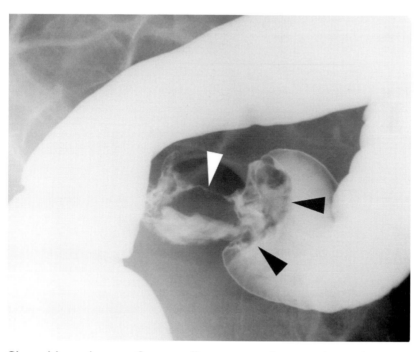

Sigmoid carcinoma. Gastrograffin enema confirms an obstructing proximal sigmoid carcinoma (arrowheads). Only a thin 'string' of contrast is seen traversing the carcinoma.

- **MRI:** important in local staging of rectal carcinoma, as it is more sensitive than CT in staging pelvic malignancy. Contrast-enhanced MRI is more sensitive than CT in detecting hepatic metastases.
- **Fluoroscopic stenting:** in inoperable disease, a palliative fluoroscopically placed expanding stent can be used to preempt or treat LBO.

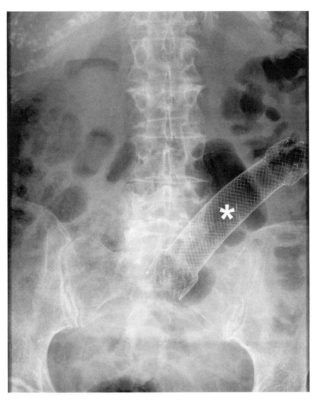

Fluoroscopic stenting. Following the insertion of an expandable metal stent (asterisk) to relieve the obstruction, the proximal bowel is decompressed.

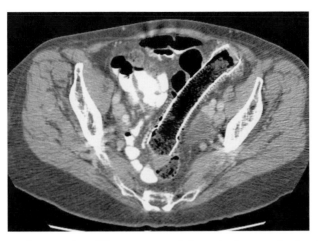

Fluoroscopic stenting. The position of the colonic stent is clearly assessable on CT.

Colonic diverticulitis

Clinical characteristics

- Diverticular disease of the colon occurs when overactive smooth muscle causes herniation of the mucosal and submucosal layers of the colon through the muscle layers. Predominantly seen within the sigmoid colon, although diverticular disease may be present anywhere within the colon.
- Colonic diverticular disease is very common in Western societies where the diet is low in roughage. Approximately 50% of those over 60 will be affected. Up to a quarter may suffer from diverticulitis.
- Diverticulitis occurs when a colonic diverticulum becomes inflamed, often by a faecolith. This presents with abdominal pain, usually in the LIF, fever and a raised WBC.
- Complications include perforation, abscess formation and fistula formation into adjacent structures, such as the uterus or bladder.
- Treatment is often conservative with antibiotic therapy, but surgery or radiological intervention, such as percutaneous abscess drainage, may be required.

Radiological features

- **AXR:** plain films may demonstrate a localised ileus, gas in a fistula or abscess, or occasionally a pneumoperitoneum.
- **Barium enema:** demonstrates colonic diverticula very well and may also demonstrate complications such as fistulae, perforation and abscesseses. The lumen of the colon affected by diverticular disease is usually narrowed owing to muscular hypertrophy.
- **USS:** detects thickened bowel and fluid collections, but the diverticula themselves and small gas collections are very difficult to identify. US is generally less sensitive than CT but can be used for percutaneous drainage.

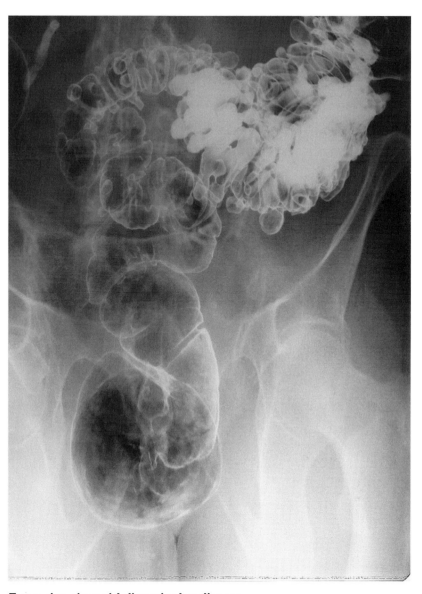

Extensive sigmoid diverticular disease.

- **CECT:** CT is the best imaging modality for visualising diverticulitis. Diverticular disease is seen as small outpouchings arising from the affected colon. These are usually gas filled, but high density within them may be from a previous barium enema or a calcified faecolith. The affected colon is often thickened by smooth muscle hypertrophy. In diverticulitis, the pericolic fat becomes 'stranded' and indistinct as a result of inflammatory oedema. Fluid- and gas-filled abscesses may be seen, as may pockets of free gas. Fistulae may be directly demonstrated or inferred through the presence of gas within adjacent involved organs such as the bladder and uterus. CT can be used to guide percutaneous drainage of fluid collections.
- It is important to remember that a carcinoma can occur within a segment of colon affected by diverticular disease, and this can lead to diagnostic confusion. Carcinoma often causes a shorter segment of bowel thickening with heaped-up margins – the so-called 'apple core' lesion seen in barium enemas.

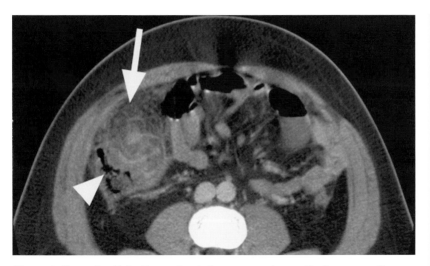

Caecal diverticulitis. Extensive inflammatory 'stranding' surrounding a thickened caecum (arrow); note the localised posterior perforation (arrowhead).

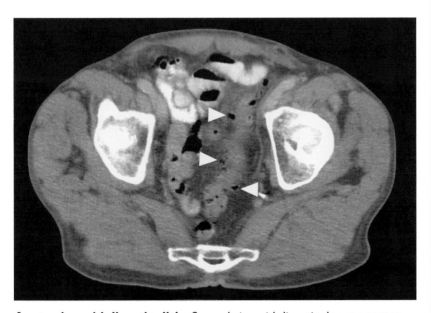

Acute sigmoid diverticulitis. Several sigmoid diverticula are present (arrowheads) and the surrounding fat is 'dirty' owing to local inflammatory change.

Colonic polyps

Adenomatous colonic polyps

Clinical characteristics

- Adenomatous colonic polyps are often asymptomatic but have the potential to undergo malignant change. Adenomatous polyps of 5–9mm have a 1% incidence of malignant change while those >2cm have an incidence of almost 50%. Polyps >10mm need to be excised.
- Symptoms include diarrhoea, abdominal pain, rectal bleeding and hypokalaemia.

Radiological features

- Endoscopic examination of the colon has the advantage of allowing biopsy and excision of any polyps, but it is an invasive procedure, and examination of the whole colon may be incomplete in a percentage of patients.
- **Barium enema:**
  - Double-contrast barium enemas have been the mainstay in colonic imaging in the past, having a false-negative rate of 7% for polyps <10mm.
  - Colonic polyps have characteristic appearances on barium enema, the main cause of diagnostic confusion being differentiation from colonic diverticula.
  - The table shows the features of colonic polyps.

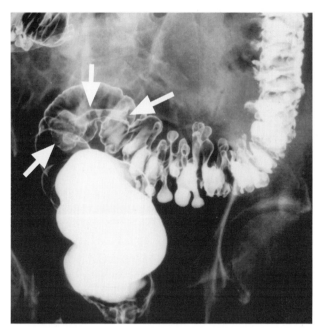

Pedunculated polyp (arrows) seen within the distal sigmoid colon.

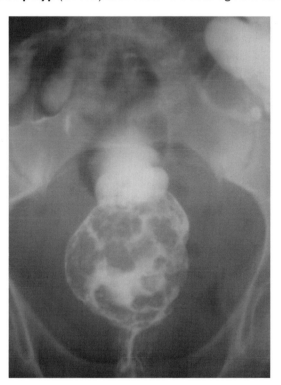

Large rectal adenoma 'carpeting' the rectum. Contrast is seen outlining
irregular filling defects within the rectum.

Features of colonic polyps on barium enemas

Feature	Characteristics
Meniscus sign	Barium forms a meniscus around the base of a polyp. When viewed en face, the inner border of the meniscus is well defined and the outer less well defined. In the en face view of a diverticulum, the outer border is the better defined.
Hat sign	The 'hat sign' results from an oblique viewing of a polyp. The barium meniscus forms the rim of the 'bowler hat', and the barium covered polyp the body of the hat
Target sign	An en face view of a pedunculated polyp will demonstrate a 'bull's eye' appearance, caused by the meniscus around the base superimposed on the view of the barium-covered head of the polyp
Increased density sign	A polyp is an intraluminal soft tissue that is of increased density compared with the gas-filled lumen in a good-quality double-contrast enema. When the polyp is coated in barium, this can be seen as a focus of increased density
Negative filling defect	Barium pools dependently and if a polyp is sitting in this pool it may be visible as a negative filling defect
Stalk sign	An oblique view of a pedunculated polyp may show the outline of the stalk as two parallel barium lines that flare slightly where the stalk merges with the mucosa. The axis of the stalk may change as the patient's orientation does during the study

- **CT pneumocolonography:**
  - Increasingly is replacing barium enema as the radiological investigation of choice. With multislice CT scanners, polyps of 5mm can be detected with high sensitivity.
  - There are a number of advantages of CT pneumocolonography over barium studies. Although the same bowel preparation is used, the study is quicker and easier for patients. It involves a slightly higher radiation dose but provides more diagnostic information, such as staging information about a colonic carcinoma or demonstrating incidental, but significant, pathology.

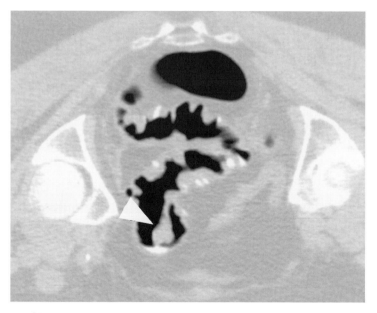

Prone CT pneumocolon. Large pedunculated polyp within the sigmoid colon (arrowhead).

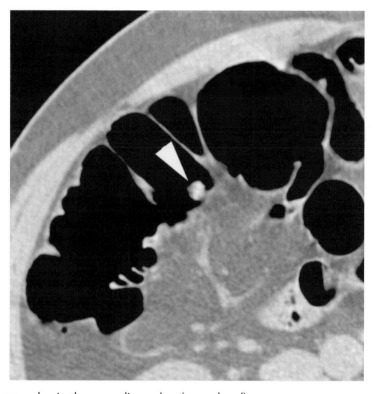

10mm polyp in the ascending colon (arrowhead).

Post-inflammatory colonic polyposis

Clinical characteristics

- This is non-neoplastic and results from the re-epithelisation of inflammatory polyps.
- Most commonly seen in UC but can be seen after ischaemic or infective colitis.
- It has no malignant potential.
- The differential diagnosis includes familial polyposis.

Radiological features

- **Barium enema:** a characteristic appearance with filiform projections, attached only at their bases.

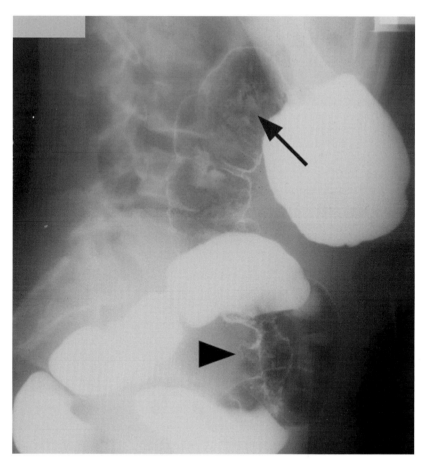

Inflammatory polyps. Barium enema in a patient with long-standing UC. Inflammatory pseudopolyps can be seen within the proximal sigmoid colon (arrow) and an irregular shouldered carcinoma within the distal sigmoid colon (arrowhead).

Crohn's disease

Clinical characteristics

- An inflammatory condition that can affect any portion of the GI tract. Skip lesions (normal areas between affected ones) are typical and help to distinguish colonic Crohn's disease from UC.
- The terminal ileum is the commonest site affected.
- The inflammation can affect all histological layers of the GI tract.
- Presentation may include weight loss, recurrent diarrhoea, anaemia, abdominal pain, peri-anal fistulae, abscesses and malabsorption.
- Complications include fistulae and abscess formation, stenosis, SBO, adenocarcinoma and lymphoma.
- The differential includes UC, enteric TB, *Yersiniae* infection, lymphoma and radiation ileitis.

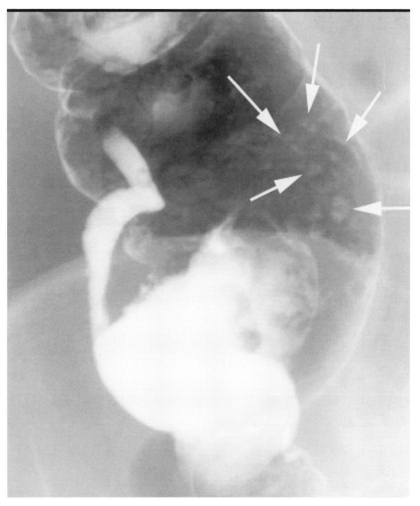

Early Crohn's colitis. Multiple shallow aphthous ulcers within the caecum (arrows).

Radiological features

- **AXR:** may demonstrate bowel wall thickening, related to inflammatory change, as well as complications such as perforation, toxic megacolon and abscess formation. However these changes are non-specific.
- **USS:** as Crohn's disease is a chronic condition that often affects young patients, repeated high-dose radiation studies, such as barium follow-through, raises the risks of long-term complications such as radiation-induced lymphoma. US can be used to assess for the mural thickening (>8mm) associated with active disease, in patients with known Crohn's disease, without exposing them to ionising radiation. US can also detect abscesses and guides the placement of drains.

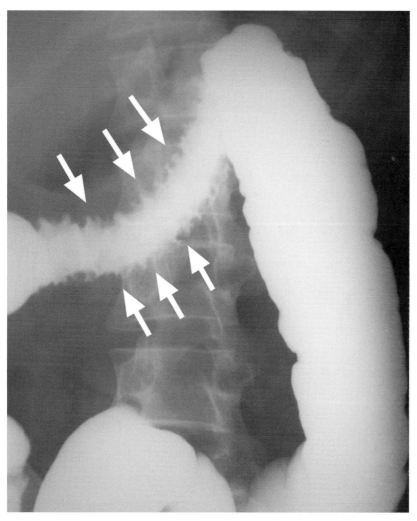

Crohn's colitis. Multiple deep 'fissuring' ulcers (arrows) seen within the distal transverse colon.

- **Barium studies:**
  - Early features include shallow aphthoid ulcers, enlargement of lymphoid nodules and thickening and distortion of the valvulae conniventes of the small bowel.
  - Later features include cobble-stoning of the mucosa, from serpiginous ulcers with intervening oedema, and rigid and straightened small-bowel loops, caused by spasm and oedema. Small-bowel loops may also appear separated owing to increased mesenteric fat and nodes. Post-inflammatory pseudopolyps may be seen. Fistulae may be demonstrated: entero-colic, entero-cutaneous or to other viscera. Pseudodiverticula are caused by outpouchings of normal bowel opposite fibrosed areas.
  - In the end stages, stenotic sections are seen with 'strings' of barium running through them. These are most common at the terminal ileum. Proximal dilated loops may be seen.

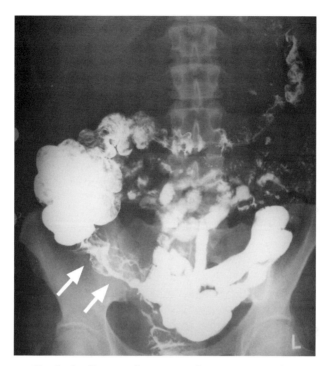

Late-stage Crohn's disease. Long irregular stricture within the terminal ileum (arrows).

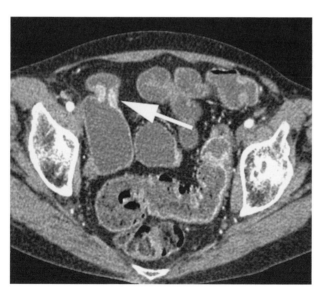

Crohn's disease by CT enterography. Short segment stricture (arrow) within the terminal ileum (arrow).

- **CT:** thickened bowel wall may show a double-halo configuration; the halo is the lumen surrounded by low-density oedematous mucosa, which in turn is surrounded by a higher density thickened and fibrotic muscularis. The increase in mesenteric fat may also be seen. Oral contrast outlines fistulae, strictures and abscesses; the latter can be drained under CT guidance.
- **MRI:** demonstrates thickened, enhancing bowel loops. T2W fat-suppressed MRI is especially useful in demonstrating the anatomy of peri-anal fistulae prior to surgery. MR enteroclysis shows promise as a radiation-free replacement for the barium follow-through and small-bowel enema.

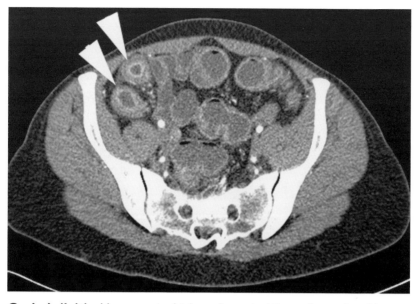

Crohn's ileitis. Hyperaemic thickened terminal ileum (arrowheads).

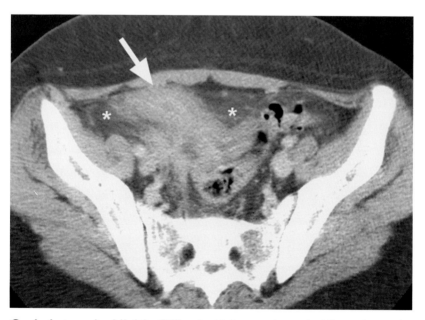

Crohn's terminal ileitis. Diffusely thickenened terminal ileum (arrow) with surrounding inflammatory stranding (asterisks).

Dermoid tumour

Clinical characteristics

- Dermoid tumour is also known as a mature cystic teratoma.
- A benign ovarian tumour that contains mature ectodermal tissues, such as fat, hair and teeth. Forms up to a quarter of ovarian tumours.
- May present as an abdominal mass or acute abdominal pain if torsion occurs.
- Often an incidental finding on imaging.
- Malignant degeneration occurs in 1–2%.

Radiological features

- **AXR:** can be diagnostic when a soft-tissue-density mass is seen within the pelvis containing focal areas of fat density, bone or teeth.
- **CT:** may show fat–fluid interfaces within the tumour. A soft-tissue nodule (Rokitansky nodule) may project into the cyst. This is made up of sebaceous material.
- **USS:** advantageous compared with CT as it incurs no radiation dose. It may demonstrate a complex mass with echo-poor cystic areas, echo-genic areas of fat, a fat–fluid level and highly echogenic areas from teeth and other calcification.
- **MRI:** again has the advantage of no ionising radiation. Although not as sensitive as CT for calcification, MRI is very sensitive for detecting the diagnostic fat within a dermoid tumour.

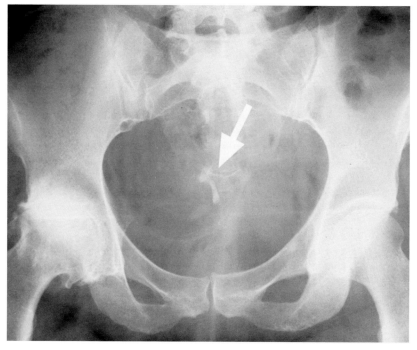

Dermoid tumour. A tooth and additional calcific debris seen within a dermoid tumour (arrow).

(A)　　　　　　　　　　　　　　(B)

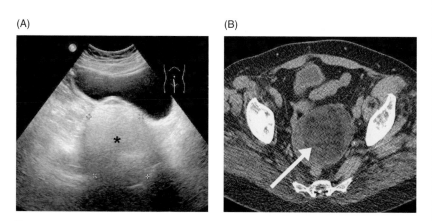

Dermoid tumour. Large echogenic fatty mass (asterisk) seen posterior to the bladder on US (A). The low-density fat within the tumour is confirmed on CT (arrow) (B).

Ectopic pregnancy

Clinical characteristics

- Ectopic pregnancy is implantation of an embryo outside the uterine cavity.
- It is associated with a history of a previous ectopic pregnancy, tubal surgery, pelvic inflammatory disease, endometriosis and use of an IUCD.
- Usually presents by the 7th week of pregnancy.
- Most (95%) occur in the fallopian tube.
- Other sites are ovarian, intra-abdominal and cervical.
- Symptoms include vaginal bleeding, abdominal pain and an adnexal mass.
- May present with hypovolaemic shock in a ruptured ectopic pregnancy.

Radiological features

- May be diagnosed by TA or TV US. The latter is more sensitive but also more invasive.
- **USS:** only specific finding by TA/TV US is visualisation of a live ectopic embryo but this is seen in less than 20% of cases. Supportive findings include no intrauterine pregnancy at 6 weeks of gestation, pelvic free fluid or hyperechoic clot, hydro- or haematosalpinx or a thickened endometrium. A pseudogestational sac may be seen – consisting of endometrial thickening with an anechoic centre composed of haemorrhage.
- Extensive intra-abdominal and pelvic haemorrhage may be seen in women with a ruptured ectopic pregnancy. This can be assessed on both US and CECT.

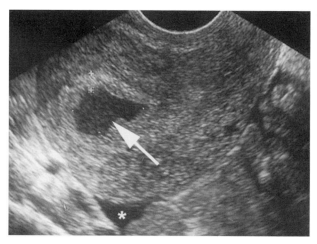

Ectopic pregnancy. Pseudogestational sac (arrow) with free fluid in the pouch of Douglas (asterisk).

(A)
(B)

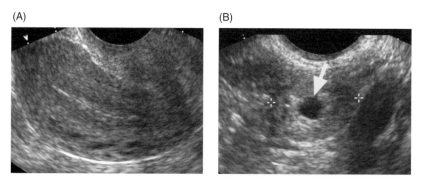

Ectopic pregnancy. The uterus (A) appears normal with no intra-uterine pregnancy identified. However an extra-uterine gestation sac is seen in the right adnexa (B).

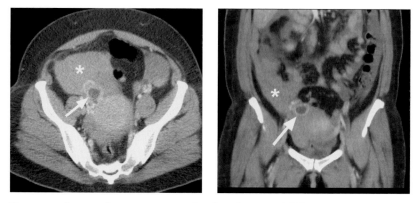

Ruptured ectopic pregnancy. Axial and coronal CT show extra-uterine gestation sac (arrow) with extensive haemoperitoneum (asterisk).

Endometrial carcinoma

- Endometrial carcinoma is the most prevalent female cancer of the genital tract and 4th most prevalent cancer in women.
- Adenocarcinoma make up 90–95%.
- Tumours of epithelial and mesenchymal origin (sarcomata) form 5–10%; such as Leiomyosarcoma, malignant mixed müllerian tumours, adenosarcomas, gestational trophoblastic tumours.
- Incidence in UK is 4900 per annum, 990 deaths annually.
- Disease of postmenopausal women; peak age 55–62 years, 75% over the age of 50 years.
- Risk factors:
  - exposure to unopposed oestrogens, such as extrinsic oestrogen therapy and tamoxifen, is common risk.
  - obesity.
  - nulliparity.
  - ovarian malfunction in polycystic ovaries.
  - late menopause.
- Other associations are:
  - diabetes mellitus.
  - smoking.
  - hypertension.
  - association with breast cancer.
- 90% arise within uterine epithelium: 90% of these are well-differentiated adenocarcinoma (grade I).
- Endometrial cancer arises in the glandular component of endometrial epithelium.
- Grows as a polypoid mass within the endometrial cavity, producing ulceration and vaginal bleeding.
- Spread is by:
  - direct invasion of the myometrium and extension through to the serosa.
  - direct invasion of parametrium with serosal seeding.
  - direct extension down endocervical canal.
- Uterus has a rich blood and lymphatic supply, a common route of spread.
- Lymph node and haematogeneous metastases are common:
  - upper uterine body tumours spread to common iliac and para-aortic nodes.
  - mid and lower uterine body tumours spread to parametrial, para-cervical and obturator nodes.
  - metastases via round ligament and vaginal extension produce inguinal adenopathy.
- Distant spread is to bone, lungs, liver and brain.

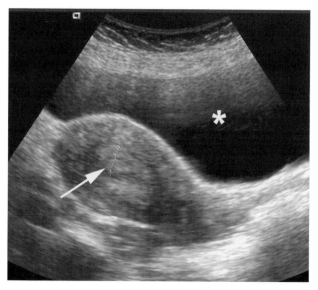

Endometrial carcinoma. TA US of the pelvis demonstrating abnormal endometrial thickening (arrow). Asterisk indicates the bladder.

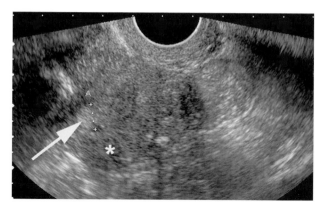

Endometrial carcinoma. TV US of the pelvis demonstrating abnormal endometrial thickening (arrow/calipers). Asterisk indicates the body of uterus.

Clinical characteristics

- Usually presents with intermenstrual/postmenopausal vaginal bleeding.
- Occasionally in advanced disease, presents with sequelae of distant spread to target organs or peritoneum.
- Rarely presents with an abdominal (uterine) mass.

Radiological features

- FIGO classification used to stage uterine cancer:
  Stage I: tumour confined to endometrium or myometrium (A–C).
  Stage II: invasion of cervix (A–B).
  Stage III: invasion of serosa, adnexae (A) or vagina (B) with nodal metastases (IIIC).
  Stage IV: invasion of bladder/bowel (IVA) or distant metastases (IVB).
- Depth of myometrial invasion is the most important prognostic factor: incidence of nodal mestastases rises from 3% (stage IB) to 40% (stage IC).
- TV US, CT and MRI are all capable of assessing myometrial invasion.
- Early endometrial disease best assessed by direct visualisation and biopsy.
- Cross-sectional imaging best for more advanced disease.
- **USS (TV/TA):**
  - TV/US in the preferred modality due to greater sensitivity.
  - Increase in endometrial thickness >5mm, usually echogenic, irregular poorly defined boundary.
  - Myometrial invasion demonstrated as disruption of the normally smooth interface between the endometrium and myometrium.
  - Depth of invasion assessed by proportion of myometrium occupied by echogenic tumour.
  - Accuracy is 77–91%.
  - Cervical involvement often detected.
  - Usually superior to CT, equivalent to MRI for myometrial invasion assessment.
  - Extra-uterine and nodal spread not accurately determined.
  - Diagnostic value of Doppler blood flow measurements is controversial.
- **CECT:**
  - Demonstrates endometrial tumour as a hypodense mass in the endometrial cavity or myometrium, or fluid-filled uterus caused by endocervical canal obstruction by the tumour. Not used for local staging.
  - Capable of detecting deep myometrial invasion.
  - May show cervical extension but less accurate than TV US or MRI.
  - Accuracy of 58–76%.
  - Often cannot differentiate from benign uterine masses, so less useful in early disease.
  - Most useful for advanced disease and detection of distant metastases, pelvic extension and nodal mestastases.
- **MRI:**
  - Excellent for local staging.
  - Widening or heterogeneity of signal within endometrial canal may be only sign in stage IA carcinoma (confined to endometrium).
  - Endometrial tumour has lower signal than endometrium, and higher signal than myometrium.

(A)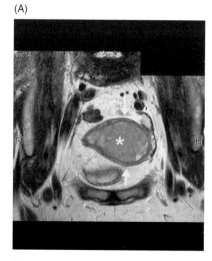

(B)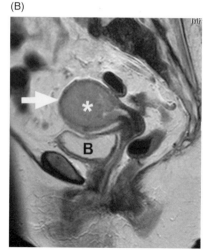

Endometrial carcinoma. Axial (A) and sagittal (B) T1 MRI of the pelvis after intravenous contrast. Abnormal enhancing soft tissue is seen expanding the endometrial cavity (asterisk). The body of uterus is markedly thinned (arrow). B, bladder.

- Disruption or absence of junctional zone implies myometrial invasion; however, junctional zone may not be visible in some post-menopausal women.
- Myometrial invasion shown as areas of relatively high signal within the low-signal myometrium.
- Contrast-enhanced T1W images clearly define zonal anatomy and improve accuracy.
- Endometrial cancer enhances more slowly than endometrium (bright on T1W) or myometrium (dark on T1W).
- Relationship of tumour to cervix is important prognostically.
- Multiple planes used to assess both longitudinal and radial tumour spread.
- Cervical epithelium is hyperintense on T2W and late post-gadolinium T1W images; disrupted in cervical extension.
- MRI is superior to TV US and CT in predicting cervical stromal invasion.
- MRI is inferior to hysteroscopy in detecting mucosal involvement.
- Overall sensitivity of MRI is 82–94% in detecting deep myometrial invasion.

Familial polyposis coli

Clinical characteristics

- An autosomal dominant condition with 80% penetrance that is characterised by a myriad of (~1000) colonic adenomatous polyps.
- The polyps develop at the age of puberty.
- Symptoms include vague abdominal pain, bloody diarrhoea and protein-losing enteropathy.
- The main complication is malignant transformation. By 20 years following diagnosis, almost 100% will have developed colonic carcinoma. There is also a lesser increase in the incidence of gastric and small-bowel malignancy.
- The treatment is total colectomy in the late teens or early twenties.

Radiological features

- Generally now diagnosed in family members by colonoscopy, but sporadic cases may present at barium enema with a myriad of small polyps forming a 'carpet' throughout the colon. There may be evidence of carcinoma, often with more than one synchronous tumour.
- **CT colonography** can reliably detect polyps of 5 mm and smaller but represents a significant radiation dose in patients who are usually in their teens at the time of investigation.

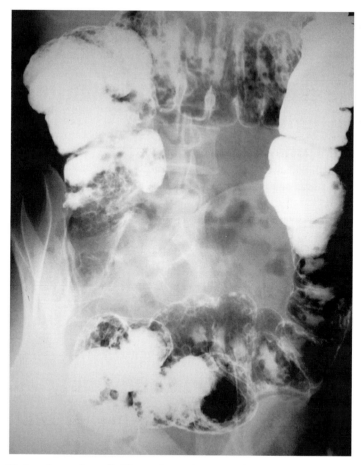

Familial polyposis coli. The colon is 'carpeted' in multiple small polyps.

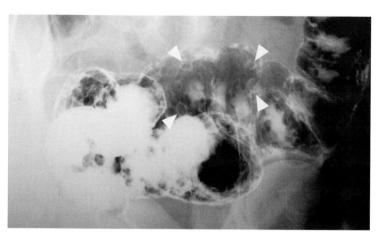

Familial polyposis coli (same patient; enlarged view of the sigmoid colon). Multiple polyps are clearly evident (arrowheads).

Fistulae

Clinical characteristics

- A fistula is an abnormal communication between two epithelialised surfaces. Examples include biliary–enteric, entero–cutaneous, aorto–enteric, entero–vesical, ano–rectal, vesico–colic.
- The causes include trauma, surgical complication, infection and inflammation, for example secondary to inflammatory bowel disease and diverticular disease.
- Clinical presentation will depend on the type of fistula.

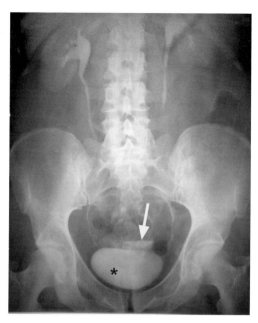

Vesico-vaginal fistula. Film from an IVU series. Contrast within the bladder (asterisk) is seen within the vaginal vault (arrow).

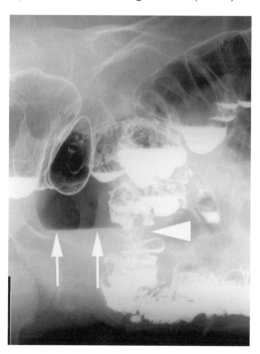

Colo-vesical fistula. Barium enema decubitus film (left side down) shows diverticular stricture (arrowhead) and an air–barium level within the bladder (arrows).

Radiological features

- Imaging of a fistula is aimed at identifying its exact path and any underlying disease to aid surgical repair.
- **AXR:**
  - Plain radiography generally is not helpful in diagnosing fistulae.
- **Fluoroscopy** following the instillation of iodinated contrast into a cutaneous fistula (fistulogram) can be useful to demonstrate the tract.
- **Barium:** similarly barium in the bowel, either as a small bowel follow-through or barium enema, or water-soluble contrast in the bladder as a cystogram, may be used to demonstrate a fistula.
  - Nonetheless, it is important to be aware that the fistulous tract may be very small and, therefore, difficult to see on these studies.
  - Despite this, such studies may be of use in delineating the extent of underlying bowel disease.

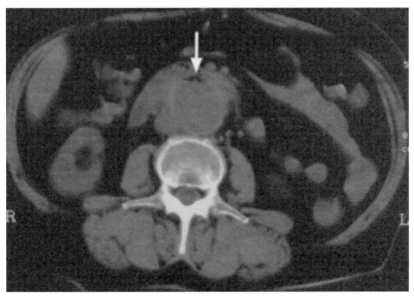

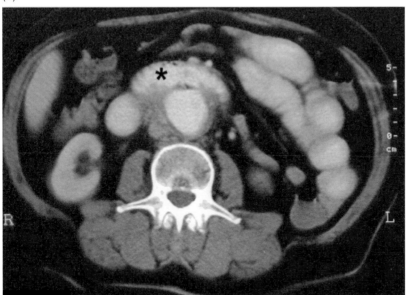

Aorto-enteric fistula. Axial CT before (A) and after (B) contrast. On the unenhanced scan, a small pocket of gas is seen along the anterior wall of the aortic graft (arrow), caused by infection. Following contrast, enhancement is seen within several small bowel loops (asterisk) from a fistula.

- **US, CT and MRI:**
  - All these modalities may be of use in imaging fistulae.
  - A mass may be seen associated with the fistula, particularly when it is caused by an inflammatory condition such as diverticular disease or inflammatory bowel disease.
  - The tract may also be visible.
  - Air may be seen within the bladder in a colo-vesical fistula.
  - Usually CT is the most useful of these cross-sectional modalities.
- **Angiography:**
  - Angiography may be necessary to help to diagnose an aorto-enteric fistula between the aorta and bowel, most commonly the third or fourth part of the duodenum.
  - This usually occurs in a patient with a preexisting aortic graft who presents with an upper GI bleed, pain or a pulsatile mass.
  - Alternatively, an aorto-enteric fistula may be investigated with CT pre- and postcontrast.

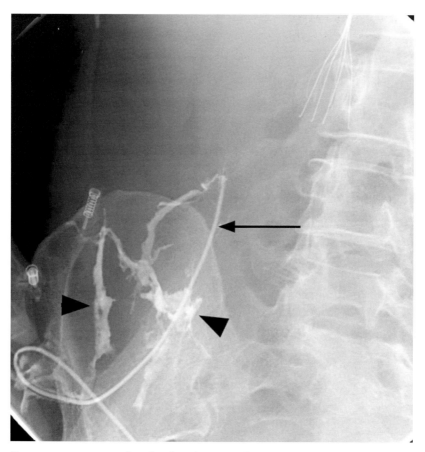

Entero-cutaneous fistula. Fistulogram where contrast is injected via a cannula though the cutaneous ostium (arrow) demonstrates a fistula to both small bowel and caecum (arrowheads). Note the presence of an IVC filter adjacent to the L₃ vertebral body.

Foreign bodies

Clinical characteristics

- Foreign bodies may appear in abdominal imaging following trauma, iatrogenic intervention, and patient ingestion or insertion – either intentionally or accidentally.
- There is a wide range of presentation, ranging from asymptomatic to *in extremis*.
- Children tend to swallow coins, marbles, disc batteries and crayons.
- Adults tend to swallow dentures, chicken and fish bones or may obstruct on a food bolus.
- Bizarre ingestions are more likely with psychiatric patients and a subgroup of prison inmates.
- Within the oesophagus there are three points of narrowing where a foreign body is likely to impact: the cricopharyngeus, at the level of the aortic arch and at the lower oesophageal sphincter.
- Once a foreign body has passed in to the stomach, there is an 80–90% chance of it passing through the GI tract.
- The main obstacle to passage through the small bowel is the ileocaecal valve.
- Complications include laceration, perforation, associated peritonitis, abscess formation and infection. Disc batteries may cause oesophageal erosion.

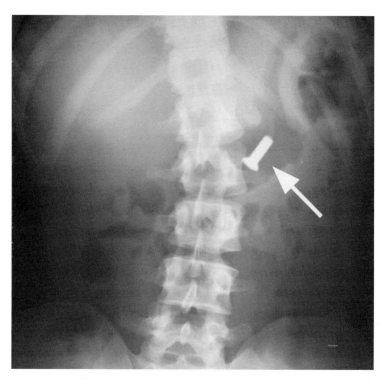

Foreign body. Swallowed screw within the stomach (arrow).

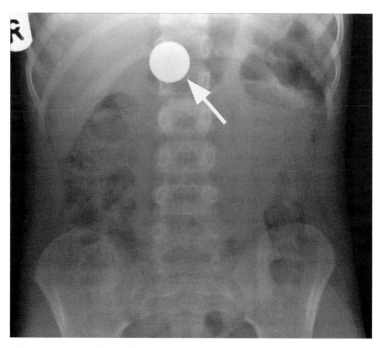

Foreign body. Swallowed coin within the stomach (arrow).

Radiological features of ingested foreign bodies

- The imaging of an ingested foreign body consists of a CXR to assess whether the body lies in the oesophagus.
- In children, this should include the neck.
- For fish and chicken bones, a soft tissue lateral radiograph of the neck is indicated.
- In adults, a lateral CXR may also be needed if the frontal radiograph is negative.
- If the foreign body has passed into the stomach, the patient can be reassured.
- Generally, AXR is not justified because of radiation dose. Two exceptions are singestion of sharp or poisonous objects, such as open safety pins or batteries.

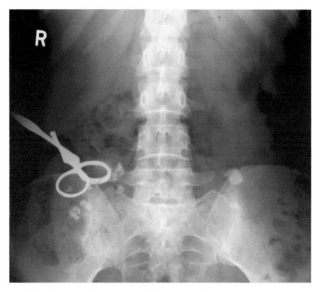

Foreign body. Retained forceps following a laparotomy.

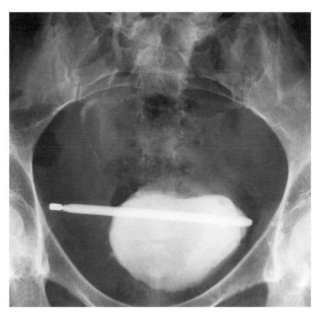

Foreign body. Mercury thermometer deliberately inserted into the bladder.

Radiological features of iatrogenic/inserted and incidental foreign bodies

- **AXR:**
  - Detects radioopaque foreign bodies, such as metallic materials and some types of glass.
  - Can be useful for checking the position of medical devices, for example the 'lost IUCD', as well as screening postoperative patients when a surgical item is unaccounted for.
  - If an unexpected foreign body is found, always consider that it may be within the patient's clothes.
  - Remember not all foreign bodies are radioopaque, for example wood.
- **USS:** initial investigation for checking whether an IUCD is within the endometrial cavity, thereby avoiding the radiation dose of an AXR.
- **CT:** useful for assessing secondary complications of foreign bodies.

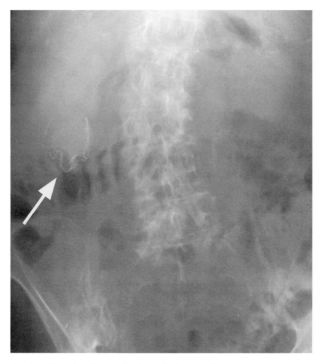

Foreign body. Retained surgical swab (arrow).

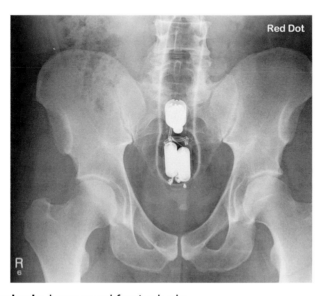

Foreign body. Large rectal foreign body.

Free intra-abdominal gas

Pneumoperitoneum

Clinical characteristics

- The aetiology of pneumoperitoneum includes perforation of a hollow viscus, through trauma, iatrogenic intervention or from inherent bowel disease, such as a perforated ulcer. Other causes include gas entering via the peritoneal surface, such as trans-abdominal biopsy or catheter placement, and via the female genital tract.
- Gas-forming peritonitis or the rupture of a gas-filled intraperitoneal abscess can also lead to a pneumoperitoneum.
- Postoperative gas takes a variable amount of time to disappear but if it remains for more than 3 days consider ongoing gas leakage.

Radiological features

- **Erect CXR:**
  - Small amounts of free gas are generally seen first in the RUQ as a single area of radiolucency lying between the right hemidiaphragm and the liver.
  - Volumes as small as 2 ml may be identified.
  - Gas may also be seen under the left hemidiaphragm.
  - Be aware that the patient should be in the erect position for at least 5 min before the CXR is taken to allow free gas to accumulate under the diaphragm.
- **Decubitus AXR:**
  - On occasion, the patient may not be able to maintain an erect position for long enough, in which case a left lateral decubitus AXR (left side down) can be helpful.
  - In this position, free gas will lie between the lateral aspect of the liver and the diaphragm.

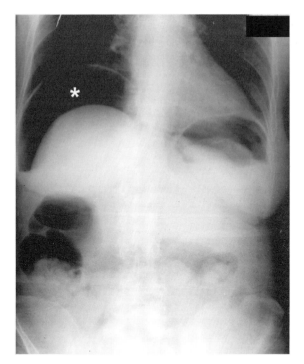

Free air under the diaphragm (asterisk).

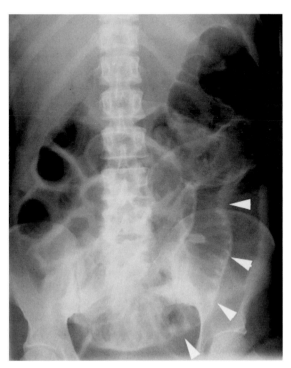

Free intra-abdominal air (Supine AXR). Note Rigler's sign (arrowheads).

- **AXR:**
  - The supine AXR can demonstrate free gas, although greater quantities are usually needed than with the erect CXR.
  - Free gas against a soft tissue surface will outline that tissue more clearly than usually seen on AXR: structures so outlined include the falciform ligament, the liver edge, the umbilical ligaments and diaphragmatic slips.
  - "Riggler's sign" (the double-wall) sign represents air within the bowel lumen outlining the inner surface, while free air outlines the outer wall.
  - Plain film pitfalls include Chilaiditi's syndrome, subdiaphragmatic fat, adjacent gas–filled bowel loops simulating Riggler's sign, subdiaphragmatic abscess, and diverticula of the stomach or duodenum.
- **CT:**
  - This is very sensitive for detecting free gas, but the radiation dose involved means that plain films remain the mainstay investigation.
  - On CT, areas of gas need to be carefully examined to establish whether they represent free or bowel gas.
  - May demonstrate likely site of perforation.
- **USS:** much less sensitive than the above techniques as differentiating free air from bowel gas is difficult.

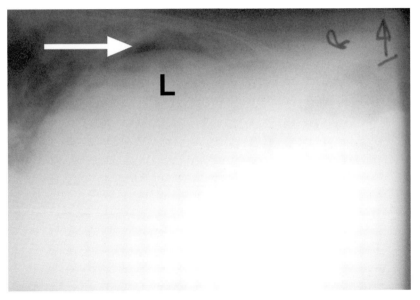

Pneumoperitoneum. Left lateral decubitus film. Note the presence of free air (arrow) between the lateral margin of the liver (L) and the rib cage.

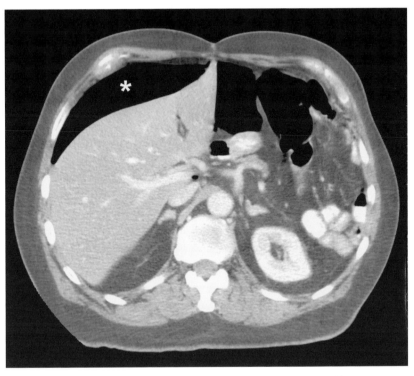

Pneumoperitoneum. Free air anterior to the liver (asterisk).

Pneumoretroperitoneum

Clinical characteristics

- Can be caused by duodenal perforation or trauma, urinary tract gas, pancreatic abscesses or gas tracking down from a pneumomediastinum.

Radiological features

- **AXR:** the presence of gas in the retropertioneum may sharply outline the kidney and psoas muscle, and streaks of gas may outline the muscle bundles.

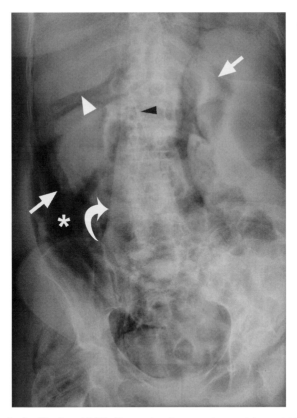

Peritoneal air (Supine AXR). Extensive intraperitoneal (asterisk) and retroperitoneal free air following ERCP. Note a biliary stent in situ (black arrowhead). The inferior margin of the liver is outlined in the intraperitoneal compartment (white arrowhead), with the kidneys (arrows) and psoas muscles (curved arrow) outlined in the retroperitoneal compartment.

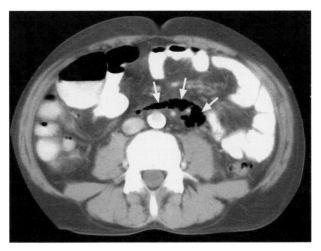

Pneumoretroperitoneum. Free air within the retroperitoneum (arrows).

Gallstones

Clinical characteristics

- Gallstones are common, affecting 10–20% of the population.
- Two main components are cholesterol and calcium bilirubinate
- There are three types of gallstone, based on their components: cholesterol, pigment and mixed, of which mixed is the most common type.
  - Cholesterol stones are caused by precipitation of supersaturated bile and occur in the Western population.
  - Pigment stones occur from excessive haemolysis, resulting in excess unconjugated bilirubin and hence precipitation of calcium bilirubinate.
- Gallstones may be present for decades without causing symptoms or complications, and usually do not require any treatment.
- Biliary colic is the result of a gallstone impacting within the cystic duct during gallbladder contraction, which then eases as the gallbladder relaxes and the stone dislodges. The pain localizes to the RUQ and epigastrium.
- Acute cholecystitis occurs when persistent obstruction of the cystic duct causes gallbladder distension and inflammation. This may progress to pus collecting within the gallbladder, known as an empyema. If the gallbladder perforates, a pericholecystic abscess may form.
- Chronic cholecystitis occurs in the setting of long-standing gallstones and results in a shrunken gallbladder with loss of function.
- *Gallbladder adenocarcinoma occurs in patients with gallstones, but gallstones are not carcinogenic per se.*

Radiological features

- **AXR:** 30% of gallstones are calcified and 10% are visible on AXR. This is usually an incidental finding rather than a diagnostic one, owing to the high false-negative rate.
- **USS:**
  - The most important modality for imaging gallstones and their complications.
  - Patients *must* be fasted to avoid gallbladder contraction, thereby reducing false-negative investigations.
  - Gallstones appear as echogenic foci, with posterior acoustic shadowing, that move within the gallbladder when the patient is turned.

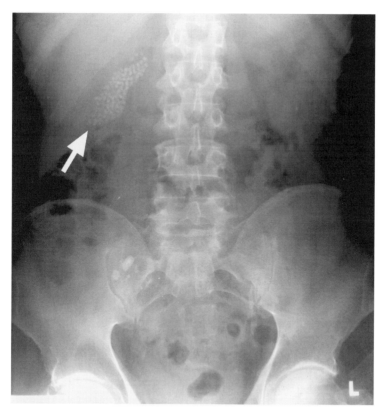

Multiple small gallstones (arrow).

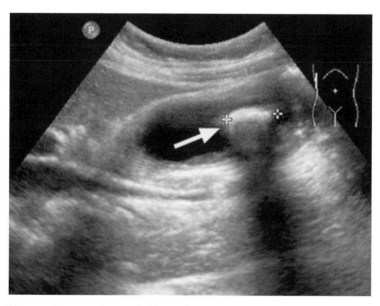

Solitary gallstone (arrow). Note the posterior acoustic shadowing.

- **Fluoroscopy:** the oral cholecystogram has largely been replaced by US for the investigation of gallstones. An oral cholecystographic agent is given and AXRs are taken the following day. Gallstones appear as filling defects in the opacified gallbladder.
- **CT:**
  - Calcified gallstones have a characteristic appearance on CT but are not as clearly visualised when non-calcified.
  - Complications such as biliary obstruction and cholecystitis may also be seen, but US remains the first-line investigation.
- **ERCP:**
  - ERCP is performed by physicians or surgeons rather than radiologists. A side-viewing endoscope is used and the ampulla of Vater cannulated.
  - Stones are visualised as filling defects within the contrast-filled bile ducts.
  - Therapeutic procedures, such as sphincterotomy and removal of stones, may also be performed.
- **MRI:**
  - MRCP is an alternative when it is not possible to perform ERCP.
  - MRCP utilises heavily T2W sequences to highlight the slow-moving fluid in the biliary system.
  - Gallstones will appear as defects of low signal intensity within the high-signal-intensity bile.

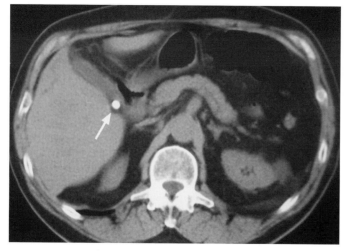

Gallstone within the neck of gallbladder (arrow).

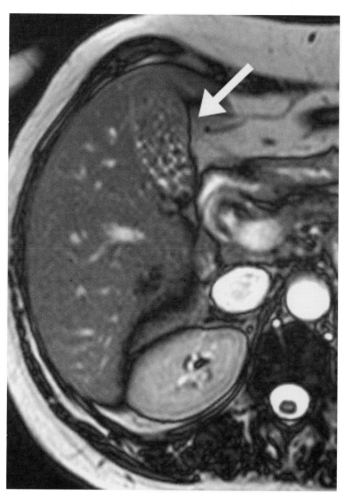

Calcified gallstones. Axial T2 MRI shows mutlpile hypointense foci seen within the gallbladder (arrow) indicating the stones.

- **NM:**
  - Iminodiacetic acid labelled with technetium-99^{m} is used to assess biliary excretion and gallbladder function (HIDA scan).
  - Failure to visualise the gallbladder by 4h, with normal bowel activity, indicates cystic duct obstruction in acute cholecystitis.
  - Has now largely been replaced by US.
- **Interventional radiology:**
  - Interventional procedures include drainage of a gallbladder empyema and PTC.
  - PTC is performed to access the biliary tree percutaneously, and involves percutaneous cannulation of the intrahepatic bile ducts via a transhepatic approach.

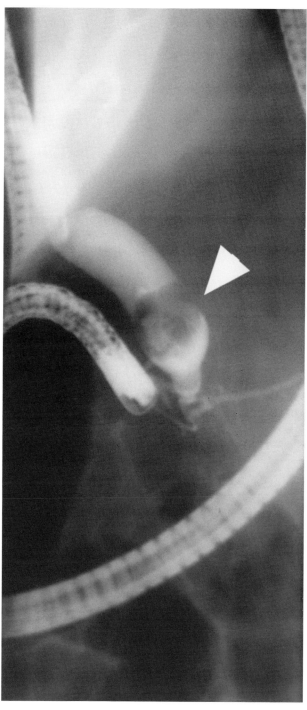

Large impacted gallstone within the distal common bile duct (arrowhead).

Hepatic masses

The differentiation of clinically significant hepatic masses from incidental, non-significant, hepatic masses is an important aspect of abdominal imaging.

Simple hepatic cysts

Clinical characteristics

- Very common incidental finding.
- Increasing incidence with advanced age.
- Associated with tuberose sclerosis and polycystic kidney disease.
- Rarely symptomatic.

Radiological features

- **USS:**
  - Investigation of choice to confirm presence of a simple cyst.
  - Well-defined, anechoic lesion with no visible wall.
  - Haemorrhage or infection may result in internal echoes.
- **CT:** fluid attenuation (0–10HU) lesion with no visible wall or enhancement
- **MRI:** very high signal on T2W imaging, low signal on T1W and no enhancement are the features of a simple cyst on MRI.

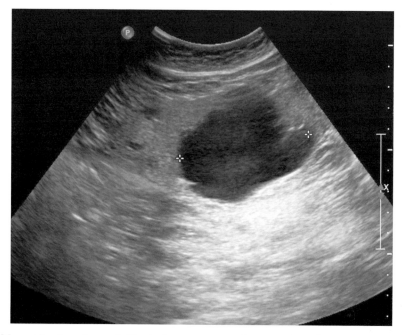

Hepatic simple cyst. Typical appearance of an anechoic lesion, demonstrating through transmission (calipers).

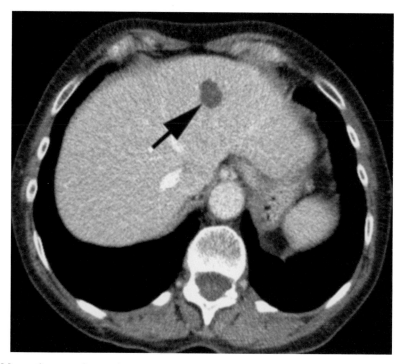

Hepatic cyst (arrow).

Hepatic haemangioma

Clinical characteristics

- A common, benign, liver lesion made up of vascular channels with slowly circulating blood.
- Most are clinically silent but larger ones may spontaneously haemorrhage or cause pain from haemangioma thrombosis.
- Kasabach–Merritt syndrome is the association of a large haemangioma and thrombocytopenia.

Radiological features

- **USS:**
  - The majority of haemangiomas are uniformly hyperechoic on US. The majority show through enhancement.
  - Some may be heterogeneous owing to scarring, fibrosis or haemorrhage.
  - Often have no Doppler signal. If detectable, the velocities are $<50\,\mathrm{cm\,s^{-1}}$
  - 90% are unchanged in US appearance on follow-up.
- **CT:**
  - Many liver lesions are investigated with a three-phase CT scan.
  - This comprises a precontrast series, an arterial phase series and a portal phase series. Occasionally delayed series are required.
  - Haemangiomas are low density on precontrast imaging. On early postcontrast, there is nodular, peripheral enhancement. Delayed imaging shows filling in from the periphery inwards. This results in complete 'in-fill' in three-quarters of haemangiomas.
  - Larger haemangiomas are more likely not to fill in completely owing to increased incidence of central scaring.
  - Small ($<1\,\mathrm{cm}$) haemangiomas may not demonstrate classical peripheral, nodular enhancement, being seen as a homogeneous enhancing lesion on early phase imaging.
  - The differential includes hypervascular metastases but these wash out on delayed imaging, and are then hypodense compared with normal hepatic parenchyma. Haemangiomas remain hyperdense on delayed images.

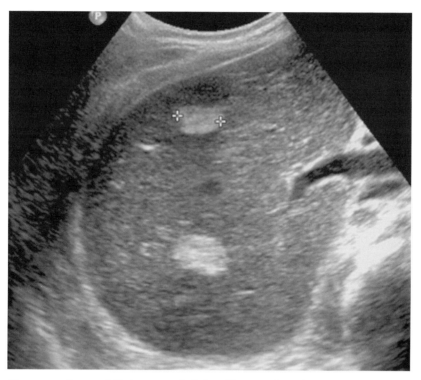

Haemangioma. US shows well-defined hyperechoic lesions.

- **MRI:**
  - MRI is increasingly used to delineate hepatic masses. It has the advantage over CT of not incurring a radiation dose, particularly important when compared with multiple-phase CT examinations.
  - Masses are well defined, sometimes with lobulated, margins. Smaller lesions are homogeneous but larger ones may be inhomogeneous because of scarring.
  - T1W sequences show iso- or hypointense lesions.
  - On T2W sequences, haemangiomas are very bright because of the slow-flowing blood. The hyperintensity characteristically remains with increasing echo times.
  - The post-gadolinium enhancement pattern mirrors that seen on CECT.

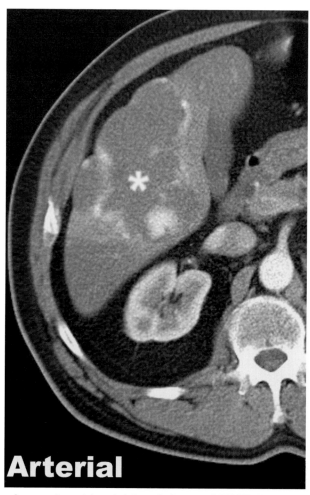

Arterial

Haemangioma. Arterial and delayed phases of CECT. Peripheral nodular enhancement is seen on this arterial phase scan, with central 'in-filling' on the delayed scan (asterisk). (See next image.)

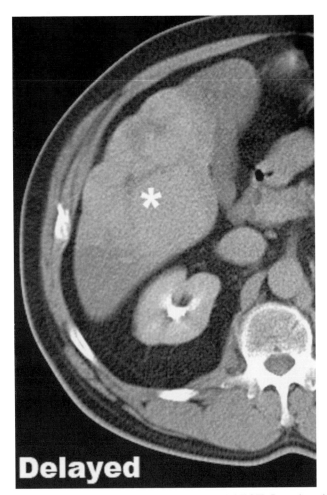

Haemangioma. Arterial and delayed phases of CECT. Peripheral nodular enhancement is seen on the arterial phase scan, with central 'in-filling' on this delayed scan (asterisk).

Hepatic adenomas

Clinical characteristics

- Benign proliferation of hepatocytes. Well defined with a pseudo-capsule of compressed normal hepatic tissue.
- May undergo fatty change, haemorrhage and necrosis.
- A condition seen almost exclusively in young females; occurs in men taking anabolic steroids.
- Hormone sensitive with an increased incidence with hormone contraception.
- Diabetes mellitus is a further risk factor.
- Growth during pregnancy may result in rupture.
- One-fifth of patients are asymptomatic.
- May present with RUQ pain from bleeding or a mass effect. Hepatomegaly may be clinically evident.
- Biopsy carries high bleeding risk.

Radiological features

- **USS:**
  - Well-defined mass of variable echogenicity.
  - The pseudo-capsule may be seen as a hypoechoic rim.
  - In larger examples, necrosis can lead to cystic regions.
- **CT:**
  - On precontrast series, adenomas are usually well defined.
  - Necrosis may lead to decreased density, while haemorrhage may lead to increased attenuation.
  - Adenomas have a vascular supply from the hepatic artery and, on arterial phase CT, show brief enhancement relative to normal hepatic tissue. Often iso- or hypodense on portal phase so may be missed if only a portal phase postcontrast series is performed.
- **MRI:**
  - As adenomas are largely composed of hepatocytes, they often have a very similar signal intensity to normal liver parenchyma on standard T1W and T2W sequences.
  - The presence of haemorrhage and intracellular fat can lead to slight hyperintensity on T1W and T2W series.
  - The presence of intracellular fat means that T1W out-of-phase sequences will lead to a drop in signal relative to liver parenchyma. **NB:** Small (<2 cm) hepatomas may also occasionally demonstrate this feature.
  - As with CECT, hepatic adenomas show transient arterial enhancement and subsequent homogeneous washout.

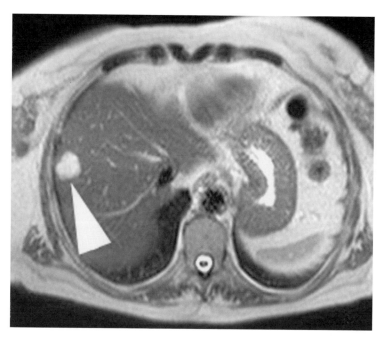

Haemangioma Axial T2W MRI shows well-defined hyperintense lesion (arrowhead); this remained hyperintense with increasing echo times.

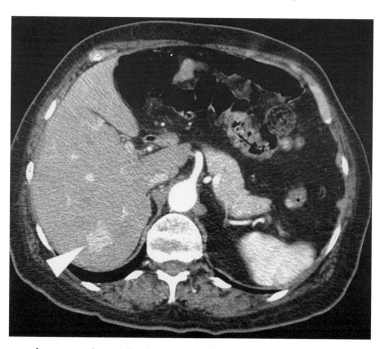

Liver adenoma. Arterial enhancement (note the intense enhancement of the aorta) of a lesion (arrowhead) within the posterior aspect of the right lobe of liver.

Focal nodular hyperplasia

Clinical characteristics

- Focal nodular hyperplasia (FNH) is a benign congenital hamartoma of the liver.
- Consists of multiple small lobules of hepatocytes. There is often a central fibrous scar with an arteriovenous malformation, producing a spoke-like pattern of radiating vessels. The lesion is non-encapsulated.
- Most are <5 cm in diameter. Often subcapsular in position and some are pedunculated.
- Not caused by oral contraceptives but may grow under the hormonal influence.
- Can be seen at any age but most commonly in the 3rd and 4th decades.
- Usually an incidental finding and are asymptomatic, although discomfort from a mass effect can occur.
- Unlike adenomas, FNHs rarely undergo necrosis or haemorrhage, and intracellular fat is rarely seen.

Radiological feature

- **USS:**
  - US may demonstrate some specific features; the mass is usually homogeneous and either hypoechoic or isoechoic to hyperechoic relative to hepatic tissue. The central scar will only be seen in one-fifth of patients.
  - Doppler studies may demonstrate the central arterial supply and the spoke-like pattern of draining vessels.
  - Shunt vessels have high velocity and arterial pulsatility.

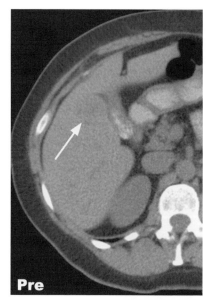
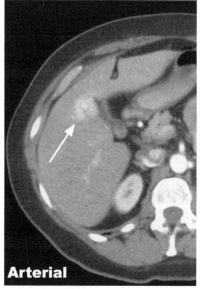
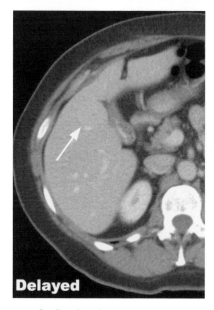

Focal nodular hyperplasia. Axial scan precontrast, arterial and delayed phase. The lesion (arrows) is slightly hypodense precontrast, with homogeneous avid enhancement during the arterial phase scan and rapid washout on the delayed scan.

- **CT:**
  - Best assessed with three-phase enhanced CT.
  - On non-enhanced CT (NECT), FNHs are slightly hypoattenuating or isoattenuating to normal liver.
  - Following contrast, there is peak enhancement at 30–60 seconds with rapid subsequent washout.
  - The central scar may enhance less on the early phase but may be hyperattenuating on delayed imaging owing to delayed washout.
- **Nuclear imaging:** sulphur colloid scans involve the uptake of isotope by the Kupffer cells of the reticular endothelial system of the liver. FNH are the only hepatic masses to contain enough of these cells to have normal or increased uptake on this imaging.
- **MRI:**
  - FNH are usually homogeneously slightly hyper- or isointense on T2W images, homogeneously hypo- or isointense on T1W images.
  - The central scar is usually hyperintense on T2W and hypointense on T1W images.
  - Following gadolinium enhancement, there is intense, homogeneous, arterial phase enhancement within the body of the FNH. This rapidly washes out to reach portal phase isointensity.
  - The scar shows late, long-lasting enhancement.

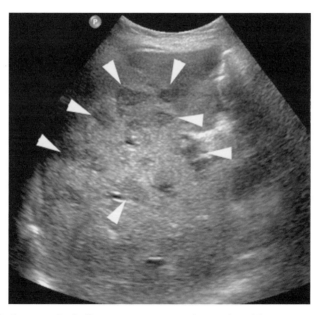

Multiple hypoechoic liver metastases (arrowheads).

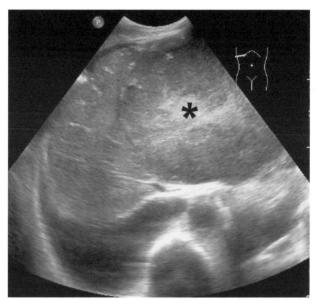

Large solid metastasis (asterisk) of mixed echogenicity. Note the presence of ascites posterior to the liver.

Hepatic metastatic deposits

Clinical characteristics

- Metastatic deposits are the most common malignant liver masses, and the liver is the second most common site of metastatic deposits after local lymph nodes.
- Common sites of origin include the colon, stomach, breast, pancreas and lung.
- Often discovered during staging of known primary tumours, but they may present with hepatomegaly, jaundice or deranged liver function tests.

Radiological features

- These can be very variable owing to the many possible primary tumours of origin.
- Mucinous adenocarcinomas, classically from colon, breast, stomach or ovary, may calcify.
- Metastases from melanoma, pancreatic islet cell tumours, thyroid carcinoma, carcinoid and renal cell carcinoma may be hypervascular.
- Metastases from stomach, pancreas, breast, lung and colon are often hypovascular.
- Hyperechoic metastases are seen in colonic carcinoma and hepatoma.
- Hypoechoic secondaries are seen in cervical carcinoma, lymphoma and pancreatic adenocarcinoma.
- **CT:**
  - Very reliable at detecting metastases, especially those <10mm.
  - Best performed with IV contrast, although a NECT may be helpful when hypervascular deposits are suspected, as these may be obscured postcontrast. NECT also helps to detect the fine calcification seen in mucinous GI secondaries – classically colonic metastases.
  - Dynamic contrast enhancement usually shows a pattern of initial, peripheral rim enhancement with a relatively hypovascular centre, leading to a 'target' appearance, with delayed washout. However many patterns of enhancement may be seen, depending on type of metastases, including non-enhancement.

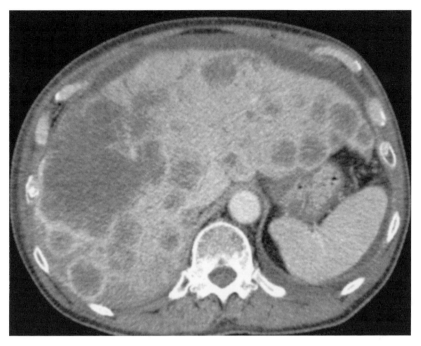

Multiple hypodense liver metastases within both lobes of the liver.

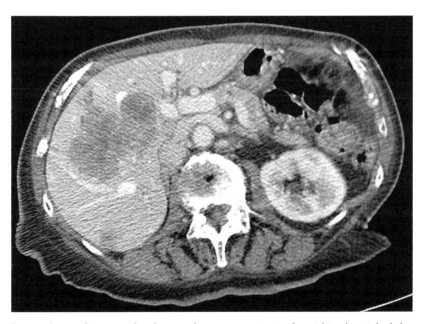

Large hypodense colonic carcinoma metastasis within the right lobe of the liver.

- **MRI:**
  - MRI is better than CT at both detecting and characterising liver masses.
  - This is important if resection or ablation of liver metastases is being considered, as the presence of multiple deposits may preclude such interventions. Conversely, MRI may establish that lesions seen on other modalities are benign.
  - Classically, metastases are slightly hypointense in T1W and hyperintense on T2W.
  - Haemorrhagic metastases may have mixed T1W and T2W signal, depending on the stage of blood product breakdown.
  - Melanin has paramagnetic properties, leading to variable hyper-and hypointensity on both T1W and T2W images in melanoma metastases.
  - Metastases from mucinous carcinomas, such as ovarian mucinous cystadenocarcinoma or mucinous carcinoma of the pancreas, may also be high on T1W images owing to their proteinaceous content.
  - Standard extracellular gadolinium enhancement patterns are similar to those of iodinated contrast enhancement in CECT.
  - Some gadolinium- and manganese-based MRI contrast agents are selectively taken up by hepatocytes, so increasing T1W parenchymal hyperintensity in those hepatic neoplasia containing hepatocytes, such as hepatic adenomas, FNHs and some well-differentiated hepatomas. However neoplasias not containing hepatocytes, such as metastatic deposits and haemangiomas, do not take up such agents. Therefore, on late (>10min) imaging, such lesions are hypointense against the contrast uptake by hepatic parenchyma. This can be helpful in detecting small deposits when liver resection or ablation is being considered.

Hepatocellular carcinoma

Clinical characteristics

- Hepatocellular carcinoma (HCC) is also known as hepatoma.
- A primary malignancy of hepatocytes.
- In the developed world, this is largely associated with liver cirrhosis.
- Other risk factors include chronic viral hepatitis, carcinogens such as aflatoxin, thorotrast, sex hormones and metabolic disorders such as Wilson's disease, haemachromatosis and α_1-antitrypsin deficiency.
- Much more common in Asia and sub-Saharan Africa.
- May present with RUQ pain, hepatomegaly, ascites, weight loss, fevers and paraneoplastic symptoms.
- Often HCCs are detected on USS.
- HCCs are associated with elevated α-fetoprotein, which is used as a screening tool in at-risk patients.

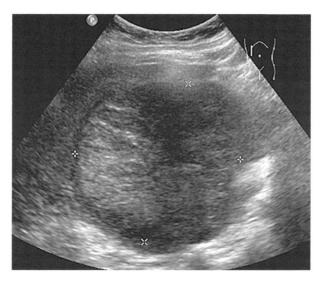

Hepatocellular carcinoma. Large solid mass within the left lobe of liver. Appearances in US are often non-specific; compare the appearance with the large metastasis pictured above.

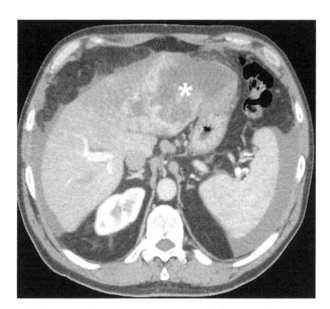

Hepatocellular carcinoma in a patient with haemochromatosis. Large irregular enhancing mass within the left lobe of liver visible on CECT; the central area of low attenuation (asterisk) represents necrosis. There is associated invasion of the left portal venous branches. Note the presence of ascites around the liver and spleen.

- Metastases may occur to the lungs, adrenal glands, bones and lymph nodes.
- Invasion of the hepatic veins can result in a Budd–Chiari syndrome. Tumour can track along the venous system, involving the IVC and right atrium.
- Portal vein invasion is also a feature.

Radiological features

- **USS:**
  - US can be used as a screening tool in at-risk patients and as an initial investigation in those with raised α-fetoprotein, but it is not specific.
  - HCCs may be focal, where a discrete mass can be seen. These may be of variable echogenicity, especially in larger HCCs when haemorrhage and necrosis are seen.
  - HCC is a vascular tumour and Doppler studies may demonstrate high velocities.
  - Invasion of venous structures can be seen.
  - Diffuse HCC is poorly defined and may be difficult to detect on US, as the subtle changes in echogenicity are difficult to differentiate against the coarse echotexture often seen in cirrhosis.
  - HCCs usually occur in cirrhotic livers where cirrhotic nodules are common. However cirrhotic nodules are rarely seen on US and any focal lesion should be considered highly suspicious.
- **CT:**
  - Detects two-thirds of HCCs in cirrhotic livers and more in non-cirrhotic livers.
  - May be focal, usually poorly defined or diffusely infiltrating. Multifocal lesions are well recognised.
  - Usually hypodense on pre-enhancement imaging; 10% may show calcification.
  - Arterial enhancement shows a heterogeneous pattern, although lesions < 1.5 cm may show homogeneous enhancement.
  - Necrotic, non-enhancing areas may be seen.
  - On delayed portal phase scans, the tumour is usually of low attenuation compared with the liver parenchyma.
  - Involvement and occlusion of the portal and/or hepatic venous systems may be demonstrated, as may areas of poorly perfused liver secondary to venous compromise.
  - Metastatic deposits, ascites and the extent of any vascular involvement can all be assessed on CT.

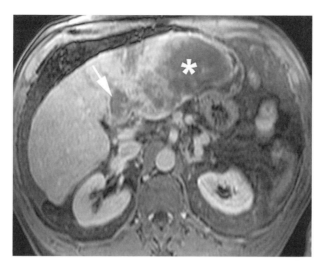

Hepatocellular carcinoma. Axial T1 fat-saturated image postcontrast from the same patient as on CT this demonstrates an irregular enhancing necrotic mass within the left lobe (asterisk) with portal vein invasion (arrow).

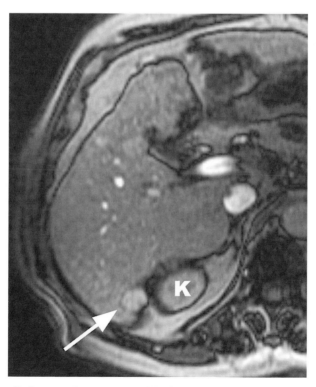

Hepatocellular carcinoma pre-ablation. Portal phase T1W MR post-gadolinium demonstrating a small mass (arrow) adjacent to the upper pole of the right kidney (K). Note the irregular liver outline in keeping with cirrhosis.

- **MRI:**
  - More sensitive than CT for the detection of HCCs.
  - The signal characteristics vary but classically the lesions are hypointense on T1W and mildly hyperintense on T2W. Hyperintensity on T1W is a known feature, caused by the presence of intracellular fat, and is associated with early, well-differentiated HCCs with a better prognosis.
  - Arterial phase gadolinium enhancement is the most sensitive sequence for hepatomas. They demonstrate diffuse heterogeneous enhancement, although, as with CECT, small lesions may enhance homogeneously. In contrast, metastatic deposits classically show peripheral, rather than diffuse, early enhancement.
  - On delayed (2 min post-injection) imaging, HCCs are usually hypointense in comparison with hepatic tissue. There may be an enhancing psuedocapsule surrounding the HCC during the late enhancement phase.
  - Diffusely infiltrating HCC is seen as mottled areas of T2W hyperintensity and early gadolinium enhancement.
  - MRI can detect metastatic deposits and assess the extent of venous complications.
  - The presence of hepatocytes means HCCs take up liver-specific contrast agents, unlike metastatic deposits.
  - There are a number of other mass lesions seen in cirrhotic livers.

    - Regenerative nodules are not neoplastic but represent local hepatocyte proliferation. These tend to be <1.5 cm in diameter, are generally iso- or slightly hypointense in T1W and T2W sequences and show no significant enhancement post-gadolinium.
    - Dysplastic nodules represent adenomatous hyperplasia and are premalignant, often developing into HCCs. Both mildly dysplastic nodules and severely dysplastic ones are usually <1.5 cm and may be mildly hypo- or hyperintense on both T1W and T2W images. The mildly dysplastic nodules demonstrate only minimal enhancement, while severely dysplastic ones demonstrate intense, but homogeneous enhancement.

Radiological interventions in hepatic masses

- As well as the use of cross-sectional imaging to obtain accurate tissue samples from liver lesions, there has been an increase in radiologically supported therapies.
- Percutaneous ablations of individual metastatic deposits and HCCs using chemical or thermal ablation have had encouraging results compared with hepatic resection.
- Ablations are performed under CT, US or MRI. One advantage of using MRI combined with thermal ablation is that changes in the signal of tissues, as their temperatures change, means real-time mapping of the burn can be performed, resulting in a more accurate ablation.
- In the future, focused high-intensity US may be used to ablate hepatic masses in a truly non-invasive manner.

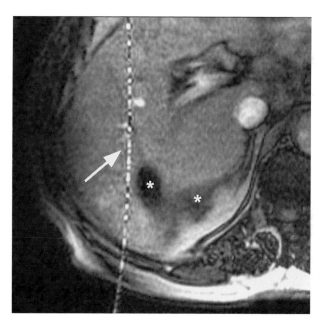

Hepatocellular carcinoma post-ablation. The ablation film is a real-time T1 image. The faint low signal line running obliquely through the liver (arrow) is the sheath containing the laser fibre. The posteromedial area of very low signal (asterisk) is the thermal burn in the carcinoma.

Herniae of the abdomen and pelvis

Hiatus hernia

Clinical characteristics

- The oesphagus normally passes through the diaphragm at the level of the 10th thoracic vertebra, and the phrenico-oesphageal membrane fixes the oesophagus to the surrounding diaphragm.
- When this membrane is deficient, a hiatus hernia occurs.
- Hiatus hernia is common and the prevalence increases with age.
- Although the majority of hiatus herniae are small, they can be very large with the entire stomach lying in the thorax.
- There are two types of hiatus hernia: sliding and paraoesophageal:
  - Sliding is by far the most common type when the gastro-oesophageal junction slides through the hiatus.
  - In paraoesophageal herniae, the gastro-oesophageal junction is in the normal position and the proximal stomach moves into the thorax, where it usually lies to the left of the oesophagus in the posterior mediastinum.
- Sliding herniae are more likely to vary in their size and position and are more commonly associated with gastro-oesophageal reflux.
- Paraoesophageal herniae are more prone to incarceration and, rarely, volvulus, and reflux is not always an association.
- Hiatus herniae are frequently asymptomatic but associated gastro-oesophageal reflux may cause dyspepsia.
- Chronic gastro-oesophageal reflux can result in Barrett's oesophagus, which is the development of columnar epithelium in the lower oesophagus; this results in a much higher risk of adenocarcinoma of the oesophagus.

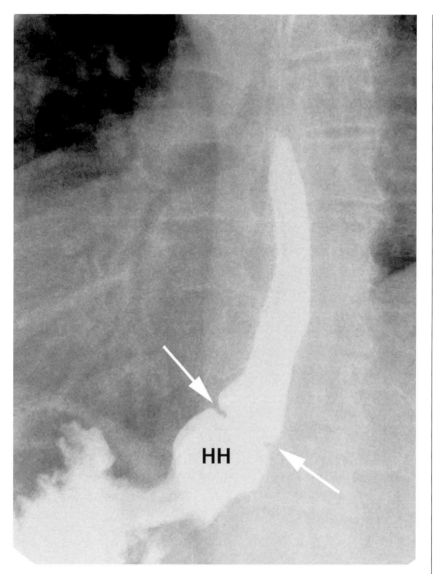

Sliding hiatus hernia (HH) with a prominent Schatzki ring (arrows).

Radiological features

- **Plain X-ray:** hiatus hernia is often diagnosed on chest radiography by the presence of a mass behind the heart, with or without an air–fluid level dependent on the patient's position.
- **Upper GI tract barium study:**
  - This is the radiological study of choice for diagnosing a hiatus hernia.
  - A double-contrast study is performed using barium and gas to coat and distend the oesophagus and stomach.
  - A sliding hiatus hernia is more easily diagnosed by endoscopy than barium study as the key feature is identification of the squamocolumnar mucosal junction, which should normally lie at 40 cm from the incisor teeth. A sliding hiatus hernia is diagnosed if the squamocolumnar junction is seen at 38 cm or less (depending on patient height).
  - The mucosal junction is more difficult to visualise on barium study and, therefore, secondary features are relied on. These features include the Schatzki, or B, ring, which is seen as a circumferential indentation in the distal oesophagus on the barium study and marks the site of the squamocolumnar junction.
  - Other features are the incisural notch, which is an incomplete ring marking the site of the mucosal junction, and the diameter of the hiatus being larger than the distal thoracic oesophagus.
  - The less-common paraoesophageal hernia is more readily seen on barium study as it does not depend upon the identification of the mucosal junction. The key feature is that the gastro–oesophageal junction lies in the abdomen.
  - When assessing for a sliding hiatus hernia, it is important to ensure maximal distension of the distal oesphagus with the patient in the prone position, and also to assess for associated gastro–oesophageal reflux with the patient tilted to the right from the supine position.
- **CT:** hiatus hernia is often an incidental finding on cross-sectional imaging, but it may also provide more detailed information of the hernial contents in a large hernia.

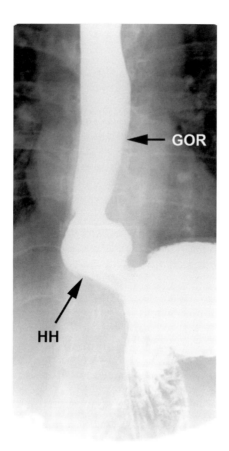

Sliding hiatus hernia (HH) with marked associated gastro-oesophageal reflux (GOR).

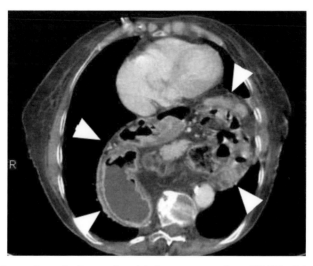

Large hiatus hernia (arrowheads) demonstrated on CECT of the thorax.

Types of abdominal and pelvic herniae

- **Epigastric:** a hernia through the fibres of the linea alba.
- **Femoral:** a hernia through the femoral canal, medial and inferior to the inguinal canal.
- **Incisional:** an iatrogenic hernia, occuring in 2–10% of all abdominal operations, secondary to breakdown of the surgical closure site from prior surgery. Recurrence rates approach 20–45% following repair.
- **Inguinal:** can be subdivided into *indirect* and *direct*. An indirect inguinal hernia passes along the inguinal canal and the hernial sac may or may not be limited to the inguinal canal. The neck of the sac lies lateral to the inferior epigastric artery. A direct inguinal hernia passes directly forward through the defect in the posterior wall of the inguinal canal, and the neck of the hernia lies medial to the inferior epigastric artery.
- **Internal:** herniation of bowel through defects in the peritoneum, omentum, mesentery or band of adhesions.
- **Lumbar:** hernia through the lumbar triangle. These tend to have a wide neck.
- **Obturator:** the hernia passes through the obturator foramen, following the path of the obturator nerves and muscles. Because of its anatomic position, this hernia presents more commonly as a bowel obstruction than as a protrusion of bowel contents.
- **Peri-umbilical:** herniation of abdominal contents through the peri-umbilical tissues.
- **Richter:** occurs when only the antemesenteric border of the bowel herniates through a fascial defect, and may lead to incarceration or strangulation of the focal herniated segment. It may occur with any of the various abdominal herniae and is particularly dangerous, as the strangulated bowel may be reduced spontaneously, leading to perforation and peritonitis.
- **Spigelian**: this rare form of abdominal wall hernia occurs through the semilunar line along the lateral aspect of the rectus sheath.
- **Umbilical**: herniation of abdominal contents through the umbilicus.

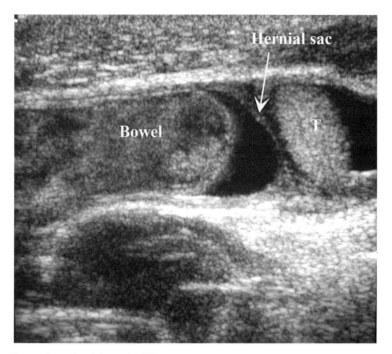

Indirect inguinal hernia. T, testis.

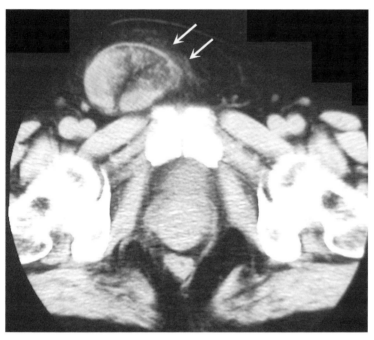

Strangulated right inguinal hernia. Note the 'stranding' in the subcutaneous fat (arrows) as a result of local ischaemia.

Clinical characteristics

- The clinical presentation of a hernia depends upon the site, size and hernial sac contents. Complications include incarceration, irreducibility, obstruction and strangulation.

Radiological features

- **Plain X-Ray:** not usually the modality of choice for diagnosing herniae; however, it is of use when bowel obstruction, secondary to a hernia, is suspected. Occasionally identified incidentally on a barium study.
- **USS:** useful to localise herniae and for differentiating from other causes of a palpable lump such as solid masses or a haematoma.
- **CT and MRI:** although US can provide good resolution of many superficial herniae, CT may provide more information regarding internal herniae.

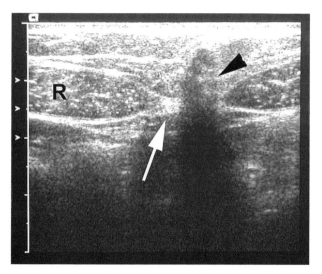

Epigastric hernia. Herniation of omental fat (arrowhead) through the linea alba (arrow).

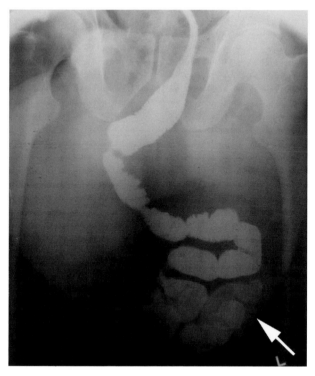

Large indirect left inguinal hernia containing multiple loops of small bowel (arrow).

- **Herniography/herniogram:**
  - This technique is less frequently used now as there are other less-invasive modalities available.
  - A spinal needle is introduced into the peritoneal cavity and radiographic contrast injected.
  - The patient is asked to cough and perform the valsalva manoeuvre to demonstrate contrast in the hernial sac.

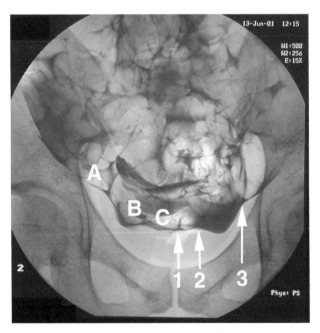

Herniogram following installation of water soluble contrast into the peritoneal cavity. **Peritoneal indentations and fossae of the anterior abdominal wall and their relation to the sites of groin hernia.**
1, median umbilical ligament (obliterated urachus); 2, medial umbilical ligament (obliterated umbilical arteries); 3, lateral umbilical ligament (containing inferior epigastric arteries). Sites of possible herniae: A, lateral fossa (indirect inguinal hernia); B, medial fossa (direct inguinal hernia); C, supravesical fossa (supravesical hernia).

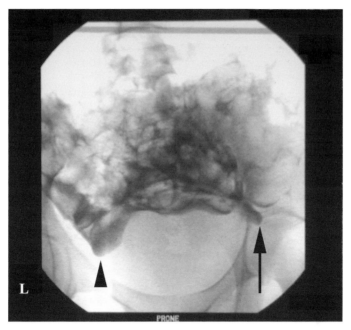

Herniogram. Direct (arrowhead) and indirect (arrow) inguinal hernia.

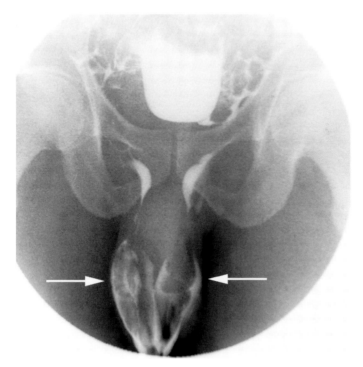

Herniogram. Bilateral indirect inguinal hernia caused by the presence of patent processus vaginalis bilaterally (arrows).

Intussusception

- Invagination or prolapse of a segment of intestinal tract (= intussusceptum) into the lumen of the adjacent intestine (= intussuscipiens)
- 90% are ileocolic and ileoileocolic.
- In adults, the majority are caused by a pathological lead point.

Paediatric intussusception

Clinical characteristics

- In 90% of all paediatric intussusceptions there is no pathological lead point and they are thought to be associated with lymphoid hyperplasia in Peyer's patches of the ileum.
- In the remaining 10%, the lead point is:
  - Meckel's diverticulum (most common lead point)
  - polyp or other tumour
  - duplication cyst
- Intussusception usually occurs in the first 2 years and rarely in neonates.
- The patient presents with severe colicky pain and vomiting. Initial stools passed at the start of symptoms are unremarkable; blood and mucus ('redcurrant jelly') stools are passed after 24h or so.
- On examination, there may be a palpable sausage-shaped mass, most often in the upper abdomen.

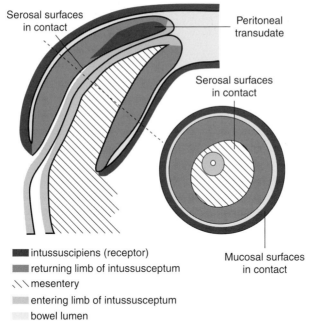

Serosal surfaces in contact

Peritoneal transudate

Serosal surfaces in contact

■ intussuscipiens (receptor)
■ returning limb of intussusceptum
\\ mesentery
■ entering limb of intussusceptum
░ bowel lumen

Mucosal surfaces in contact

Intussusception.

Radiological features

- **AXR:** film is normal in 50%. A soft-tissue mass or intraluminal filling defect, in a partially air-filled bowel loop (commonly at hepatic flexure), may be seen.
- **USS:** a 'target sign' may be seen, appearing as concentric alternating echogenic and echo-poor rings, representing compressed mucosal and serosal surfaces and oedematous bowel wall, respectively. Colour Doppler shows blood vessels dragged in between the entering and exiting layers of the intussusception. Absence of blood flow indicates devitalised bowel segments.
- **Antegrade barium study:** contraindicated in perforation. Barium examinations have been generally superseded by US. May show a 'coiled spring' appearance with a beak-like distal string of barium as it runs through the central column.
- **Barium enema:** contraindicated in perforation. Water soluble contrast enemas may demonstrate a convex intraluminal mass, representing the intussusceptum, surrounded by contrast. The 'coiled spring' sign is seen as contrast flows over the oedematous fold of the reflected intussusceptum.

Radiological management

- An intussusception can be reduced radiologically under fluoroscopic guidance with barium, water-soluble contrast or air.
- Contraindications include peritonitis and shock.
- Prior to attempting reduction, the child should be resuscitated and both surgical and anaesthetic cover available.
- The pneumatic technique is preferred as it is faster and if perforation complicates the procedure the tears tend to be smaller, and hence the degree of peritoneal contamination lessened.
- Radiological reduction can also be attempted under US guidance using saline.
- The complication rate for radiological reduction is less than 3% and includes perforation, the reduction of infarcted bowel and the non-detection of a pathological lead point.

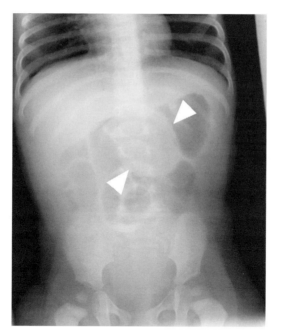

Intussusception. Soft tissue density mass within the upper abdomen (arrowheads).

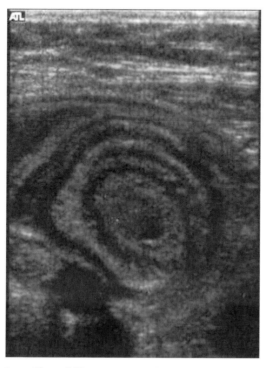

Intussusception. Classic US appearance of the 'target sign' in intussusception.

Adult intussusception

Clinical characteristrics

- Unlike in the paediatric situation, the majority, approximately 80%, have a defined lead point such as a neoplasia, inverted diverticulum, foreign body, chronic ulcers or postsurgical changes.
- Intussusceptions are the cause of approximately 15% of bowel obstructions.
- Other presentations include bloody diarrhoea, recurrent colicky abdominal pain, palpable mass and change in bowel habit.

Radiological features

- **CT:**
  - This is the imaging modality of choice. The intussusception is identified by a series of concentric rings. The central component represents the lumen and the intussusceptum wall. The middle ring is of mesenteric fat in which mesenteric vessels are usually visible. The peripheral ring is made up of the reflected intussusceptum and the intussuscipiens.
  - May also demonstrate the pathological lead point and its extent.
  - Complications such as obstruction or perforation are also well visualised.

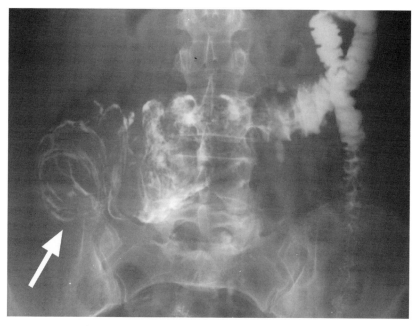

Intussusception. Single-contrast enema shows 'coiled spring' appearance (arrow) in the RUQ.

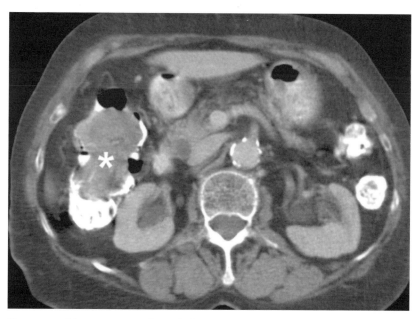

Ileocaecal intussusception. A further example that is secondary to a carcinoma (asterisk).

- **Barium studies and USS:** no longer first-line investigation, but chronic, intermittent intussusceptions may be uncovered during these investigations. The findings are similar to those in children; however, evidence of lead points is again more likely to be seen.

Management

In the adult group, management is surgical rather than radiological.

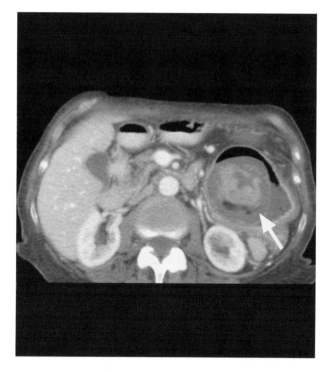

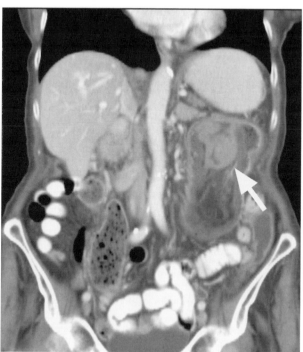

Adult intussusception. Axial CECT with coronal reformat. Large intussuscepting carcinoma within the descending colon (arrows).

Lines and devices

- It is important to be able to recognise common lines and devices used in the abdomen in order to confirm they are correctly positioned and to avoid misinterpretation.

Radiological features

- Most lines and devices are visible on AXR; however, as this is only a two-dimensional assessment, further imaging is sometimes necessary to assess the position and patency of various lines and tubes.
- US can confirm the patency of ureteric and biliary stents by documenting the absence of hydronephrosis and biliary dilatation.
- US and/or CT may be needed to assess surgical drains.
- If there is concern regarding patency of a vascular line, radiographic contrast can be directly injected into it under fluoroscopic guidance.

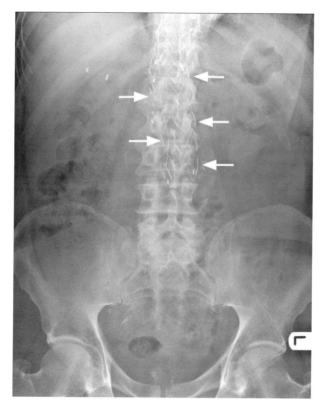

Endovascular thoraco-abdominal aortic stent seen in situ (arrows).

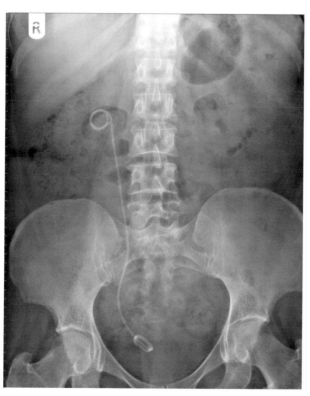

Ureteric stent. Right double 'pigtail' stent.

Types of line/device

Vascular lines

- In the neonate, umbilical arterial and venous lines are commonly used.
  - The **umbilical artery catheter** is passed via the umbilical artery into the internal iliac artery and the infrarenal aorta. On AXR, it is seen to loop down into the pelvis before travelling in a cephalic direction to the left of the midline. The tip of the line should lie either above or below the renal arteries, between T8 and T12 or L3 and L4.
  - The **umbilical vein catheter** should traverse the umbilical vein, the portal sinus (junction of left and right portal vein), ductus venosus and IVC and end in the right atrium. On the abdominal film the catheter passes in a cephalic direction from its entry point and should lie above the liver in the right atrium. The umbilical vein catheter is easily misplaced in a portal or hepatic branch and the tip is then seen projected over the liver on AXR.
- **Femoral venous lines** lie in the inguinal regions and pass in the iliac veins to the IVC.
- **Arterial stents** within the abdominal aorta and iliac arteries have a mesh-like appearance.
- **IVC filters** look like the spokes of an umbrella and lie to the right of the midline on the abdominal film.

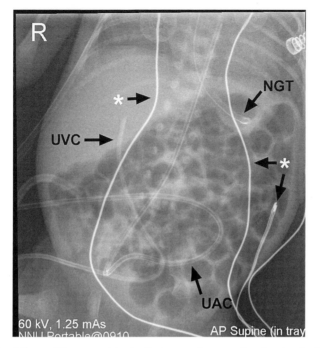

Umbilical lines. The asterisks indicate cardiac monitoring leads. NGT, nasogastric tube; UVC, umbilical venous catheter; UAC, umbilical arterial catheter.

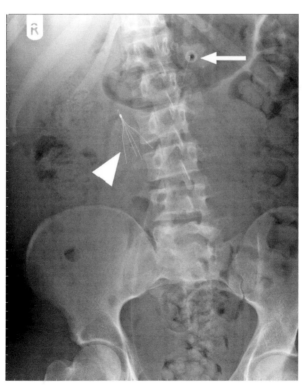

Percutaneous endoscopic gastrostomy. IVC filter (arrowhead) and tube (arrow) in situ.

Urinary tract lines

- The most commonly seen tube relating to the urinary tract on AXR is the **urinary catheter**, placed either via the urethra or the suprapubic route.
- **Ureteric stents** have curled ends and lie lateral to the transverse processes of the vertebral bodies. Transplant kidneys may also have ureteric stents that lie in the pelvis.
- **Nephrostomy** tubes placed percutaneously to drain an obstructed kidney are seen in the upper abdomen, with a coiled end in the renal angle and an external component.
- Patients with renal failure on **peritoneal dialysis** have an intra-abdominal catheter that is tunnelled under the skin before entering the abdomen and usually lies in the lower abdomen, although its position is variable.

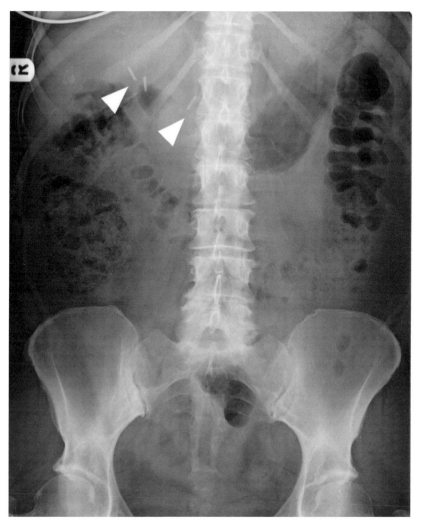

Cholecystectomy clips in the RUQ (arrowheads).

Gynaecological lines/devices

- Commonly identified devices include:
  - **intrauterine contraceptive devices** ('the coil')
  - **sterilisation clips**
  - **ring pessary:** used as conservative treatment for uterine prolapse.

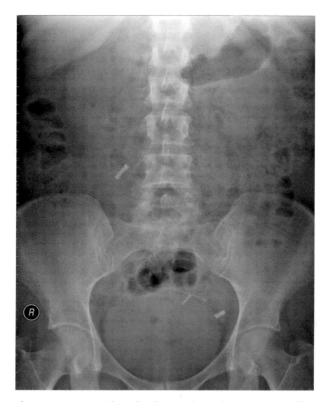

Intrauterine contraceptive device and sterilisation clips. The clip on
the right side has migrated superiorly.

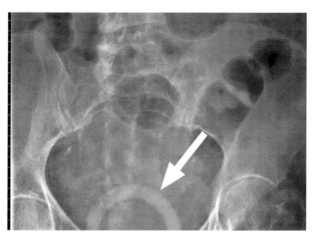

Ring pessary in situ (arrow).

Gastrointestinal tract lines

- Tubes commonly seen within the GI tract are **nasogastric** and **naso-jejunal tubes** placed for feeding. To aid identification, the tips of the tubes are radioopaque and the tips of both should lie in the LUQ. The nasojejunal tube lies more distally within the bowel and follows the C-shaped loop of the duodenum, crossing the midline into the left side of the abdomen, to lie just distal to the duodenojejunal junction.
- **Stents** placed within the biliary system, for example within the common bile duct, are visible on the abdominal film, lying in the RUQ.
- **Stoma devices**. The position of these is naturally dependent on the procedure performed.

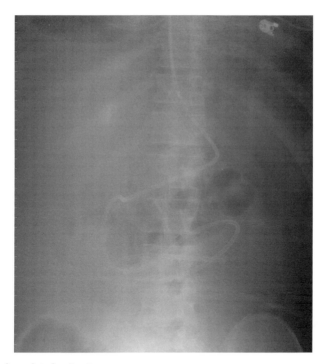

Nasojejunal tube in situ.

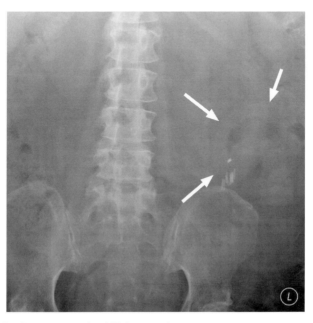

Stoma device seen in the LIF (arrows).

Surgical drains

Drainage tubes are often present in postoperative patients; the site obviously relating to the procedure performed, and hence clinical history is important when looking at the AXR.

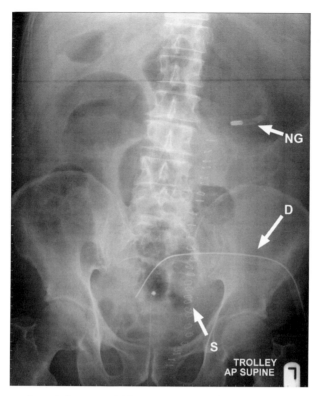

Postoperative abdomen. NG, nasogastric tube; D, surgical drain; S, surgical staples

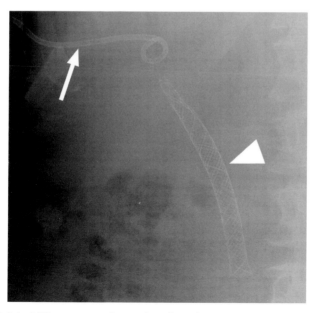

Expandable biliary stent (arrowhead) and percutaneous pigtail drainage catheter (arrow) seen in situ within the RUQ.

Lymphadenopathy

Clinical characteristics

- Lymphadenopathy can have numerous causes, which can be broadly divided into neoplastic, infective and inflammatory conditions:
  - neoplastic: lymphoma, leukaemia, metastatic cancer.
  - infective: TB, bacterial, viral, fungal.
  - inflammatory and miscellaneous: Castleman's disease, amyloid, sarcoid, mesenteric lymphadenitis.

Radiological features

- As part of the investigation of a patient with lymphadenopathy, which is apparent elsewhere, abdominal imaging may be performed.
- The main purpose is to assess the size and extent of the lymph node enlargement (i.e. regional or widespread) as well as to identify an underlying cause.
- Imaging also plays an important role in the follow-up of treated patients. Generally the smaller diameter (short axis diameter) of the node in the axial plane is recorded and regional nodal groups have different upper limits of normality. As a rule of thumb, a short axis diameter of < 1 cm is considered within normal limits, although there is overlap between benign and malignant adenopathy. However, using size as a criterion of malignancy may overlook microscopic metastases when only part of a node is involved. If a lower threshold is used to separate benign and malignant, the sensitivity increases but the specificity decreases, and when a higher threshold is applied the sensitivity drops and the specificity rises.
- **AXR:** may detect calcification within lymph nodes but overall is not helpful.
- **USS:**
  - As well as confirming that a palpable swelling is caused by lymph node enlargement, US can characterise and assess the extent of lymphadenopathy, although visualisation of the retroperitoneum can sometimes be obscured by overlying bowel gas.
  - Normal lymph nodes are usually oval and hypoechoic (dark) with hilar vascularity. They often have an echogenic fatty hilum.
  - Malignant disease alters the morphology of nodes so that they become more rounded with peripheral vascularity.
  - US is also useful for performing US-guided fine needle aspiration cytology or biopsy.

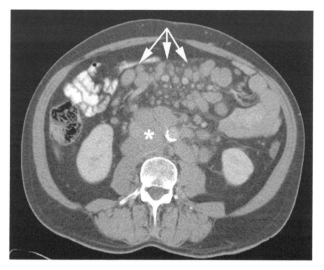

Lymphoma. Multiple large-volume mesenteric lymph nodes (arrows), with additional confluent retroperitoneal nodal masses (asterisk).

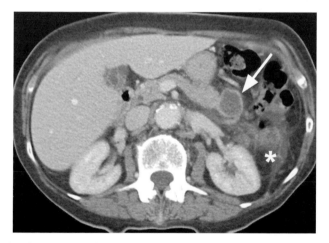

Necrotic ring-enhancing node secondary to a malignant gastric ulcer (not shown). Extensive soft tissue stranding present in the left upper quadrant from local tumour infiltration (asterisk).

- **CT:**
  - CT is particularly useful in assessing the extent of lymphadenopathy, identifying an underlying cause and any complications, for example hydronephrosis secondary to enlarged lymph nodes.
  - It is also useful as a method of following up patients known to have lymphadenopathy, after treatment.

- IV contrast is routinely given to help to differentiate lymph nodes from adjacent vessels and oral contrast or water to outline small-bowel loops.
- As on US, benign nodes may also demonstrate a fatty hilum and characteristic oval shape.
- Enlarged lymph nodes can be characterised further by their appearance. For example, tuberculous nodes typically have a low-density necrotic centre and rim enhancement after IV contrast.
- Squamous cell metastases are also typically necrotic. In contrast, lymphomatous nodes have a homogeneous appearance with minimal enhancement.
- The rare condition, Castleman's disease demonstrates marked lymph node enhancement.
- **MRI:**
  - Both normal and malignant lymph nodes have intermediate signal intensity on T1W sequences, intermediate–high on T2W sequences and enhance after IV gadolinium.
  - The same size criteria as for CT are used with the same problems.
  - There have been clinical trials using specific contrast agents for lymphoid tissue, which demonstrate improved accuracy, but these agents are not in widespread use.
- **Positron emission tomography (PET) and PET-CT:**
  - Both PET and PET–CT use the glucose analogue ^{18}F-Fluorodeoxyglucose (FDG), which is taken up by cells with an increased rate of glycolysis, as in malignant lymph nodes.
  - The disadvantage of PET is its lack of spatial resolution owing to limited anatomical information.
  - This has been improved by the combination of CT with PET to create PET-CT. The patient is scanned sequentially by the PET and CT scanners from skull base to mid-thigh and the images reconstructed and coregistered for interpretation by the radiologist.
  - PET-CT can now provide accurate anatomical information about a region of increased uptake of isotope in the PET component.
  - It is important to be aware that other conditions, such as infection, inflammation and granulomatous disease, can also demonstrate increased glycolysis. However, PET-CT has an important role in the diagnosis and staging of malignant disease.

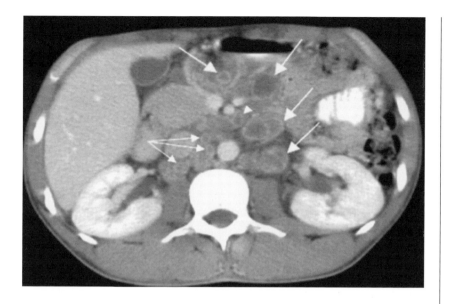

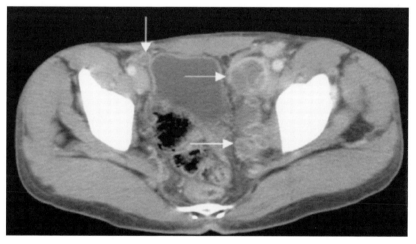

Nodal tuberculosis. Multiple abdominopelvic ring-enhancing necrotic (caseous) nodes (arrows).

Lymphoma: abdominal

Clinical characteristics

- Lymphomas are malignancies of the lymphoid tissues of the body and are broadly divided into Hodgkin's disease (HD) and non-Hodgkin lymphoma (NHL). They are a diverse group of neoplasms with some broad patterns of presentation and behaviour.
- Lymphoma accounts for 5–6% of all adult and 10% of childhood malignancies. NHL is more common than HD (60:40%); in the UK in 2001, there were 4600 deaths from NHL and 260 deaths from HD.
- HD classically shows a bimodal peak distribution: in the third decade and subsequently in the 65–75 age group. NHL is a disease of children and the elderly, with a median age at diagnosis of 65 years.
- The different behaviour of HD and NHL is reflected in their clinical staging (which is distinct from their pathological staging). While both HD and NHL are essentially diseases of lymph nodes, both may present as either localised nodal disease or as widely disseminated cancer.
- Most patients with HD present with painless asymmetrical nodal enlargement, accompanied by night sweats, fever, pruritus and weight loss in 40% (B symptoms).
  - The commonest site of nodal involvement is cervical, present in up to 80% of patients. Exclusive infradiaphragmatic disease occurs in under 10% of patients. Splenomegaly is present in about a third. HD spreads contiguously from one nodal group to the next. Primary extra-nodal HD is very rare.
- Patients with NHL also present with nodal enlargement, though in this case it is often non-contiguous and extra-nodal disease is common. Associated B symptoms occur half as often as with HD.
- HD disease is staged via the Cotswold classification, a modification of the Ann Arbor classification. Early disease is treated with radiotherapy, while more advanced disease is treated with radiotherapy and chemotherapy. Overall 10-year survival in patients treated with radiotherapy for early-stage HD is >90%.
- The prognosis in NHL is very variable. Unlike HD, histological subtype (particularly the division into low- and high-grade disease) as well as stage is the major determinant of treatment. Low-grade lymphoma is often asymptomatic and surveillance or local radiotherapy may be appropriate. In high-grade lymphoma, multidrug chemotherapy and new antibody therapies are utilised. The 10-year survival for low-grade NHL treated with radiotherapy approaches 90%.

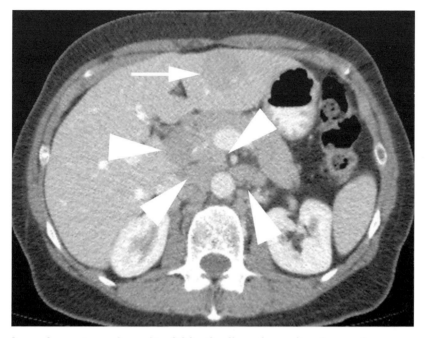

Lymphomatous deposit within the liver (arrow) and several enlarged retroperitoneal nodes (arrowheads).

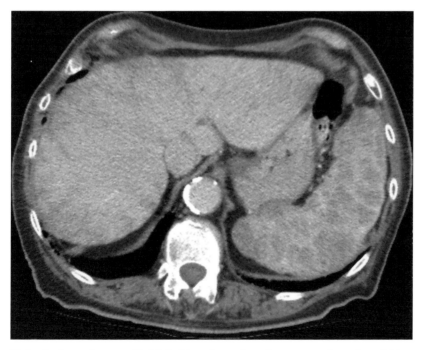

Splenic lymphoma. Multiple hypodense lymphomatous deposits within the spleen.

Radiological features

- Abdominal lymphoma may involve both nodal and extra-nodal sites. Retroperitoneal nodal involvement is present in up to 35% of patients with HD and up to 55% in NHL. Mesenteric nodes are involved in >50% of patients with NHL but only 5% in HD. In HD, coeliac, splenic hilar and porta hepatis nodes are involved in 30% of patients. Involvement of splenic nodes is invariably associated with splenic infiltration. There may be contiguous spread from mediastinal nodes in HD. In NHL, nodal involvement is often non-contiguous and may be associated with visceral involvement as well as diffuse mesenteric and omental involvement. In the pelvis, all nodal groups may be involved in both NHL and HD. Involved nodes are typically rounded, homogeneously enhancing and may form a matted nodal group particularly in NHL.
- Extra-nodal abdominal involvement in both HD and NHL may include the liver, spleen, GI tract, pancreas, genitourinary system and adrenal glands.

Liver

- Liver and invariably splenic involvement occurs in 5% of patients with HD, with 15% of patients with NHL similarly affected. Large focal areas of involvement are easily seen on CT, MRI and US as well-defined, large hypodense (on both NECT and CECT) or hypoechoic areas, but are present in only 10% of hepatic involvement. On MRI, these areas are low on T1W and high on T2W images. Imaging is insensitive to the more common diffuse microscopic involvement seen in both HD and NHL. Diffuse hepatomegaly is strongly suggestive of liver involvement.

Spleen

- The spleen is involved in 30–40% of patients with HD, usually with coexistent supradiaphragmatic disease. In 10%, it may be the only infradiaphragmatic site of disease.
- Splenomegaly, however, is an insensitive indicator of splenic involvement, with 33% of normal-sized spleens found to contain tumour at laparotomy. Splenic lymphoma may present as a solitary lesion, miliary splenic nodules or multiple low-attenuation masses on CECT and US. Optimum CECT scanning of the spleen is in the porto-venous phase of contrast enhancement. US assessment of splenic involvement is insensitive. Splenic involvement is seen in 40% of patients with NHL.
- Splenomegaly and splenic infarction are more common in NHL than HD.

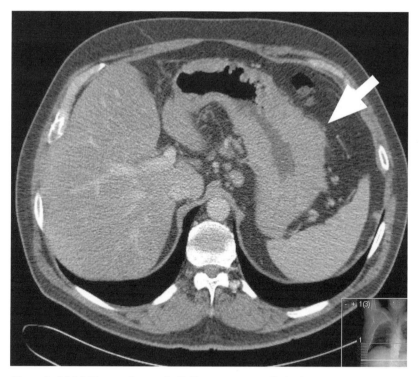

Gastric MALToma (arrow). Diffuse gastric wall thickening.

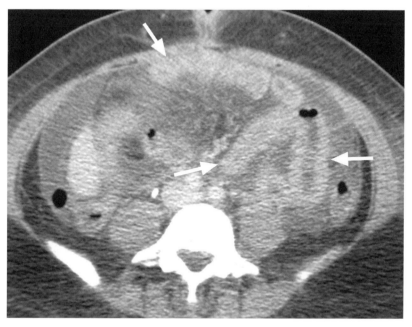

Burkitt's lymphoma. Axial section showing diffuse small-bowel wall thickening (arrows).

Gastrointestinal tract

- This is the commonest site of primary extra-nodal lymphoma in NHL.
- Involvement in HD is very rare.
- Primary lymphoma usually only affects one site. It develops from mucosa-associated lymphoid tissue (MALT tumours) and has a bimodal distribution of under 10 years and between 50 and 60 years.
- Secondary lymphoma of the GI tract is common, with stomach involvement being the most common (50%), followed by small bowel (33%), large bowel (15%) and oesophagus (1%).
- Almost 50% of patients demonstrate multiorgan abdominal disease.
- Primary lymphoma of the stomach arises in MALT. It may present as multiple nodules with central ulceration, a large fungating solitary lesion or, in 10%, diffuse gastric fold thickening. Diagnosis is best made by endoscopy but cross-sectional imaging is needed to assess the deep tissue extent, extra-gastric nodal involvement and multiorgan disease.

- **Small bowel:**
  - Lymphoma accounts for 50% of all small-bowel tumours and usually affects the terminal ileum.
  - Patients with AIDS are particularly prone to disease in this region. Multifocal disease is present in up to half.
  - As the lymphoma develops and destroys the layers of the bowel, involved areas initially produce mural thickening, leading to subsequent wall destruction, with segments of alternating constriction and dilatation.
  - Less commonly, involvement remains submucosal, leading to polyp formation and intussusception. Indeed, lymphoma is the commonest cause of intussusception in children after infancy.
  - T-cell lymphoma associated with gluten-sensitive enteropathy and α-chain disease affects the proximal small bowel and may lead to bowel perforation.
  - The small intestine may also be affected secondary to direct extension from mesenteric adenopathy, leading to encasement and displacement of affected bowel loops, peritoneal enhancement and occasionally ascites in advanced disease, which may be indistinguishable from peritoneal carcinomatosis.

- **Colon:** primary lymphoma of the large bowel is rare (0.05% of all colonic neoplasms) and usually affects the rectum and caecum, together with terminal ileum, and may present as a large mass indistinguishable from colonic carcinoma. Secondary involvement is more diffuse or segmental.

- **Oesophagus:** involvement is very unusual and when present involves the distal oesophagus resulting in a typically smooth tapered oesophagus.

(A) 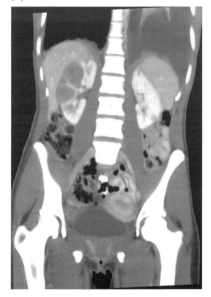 (B)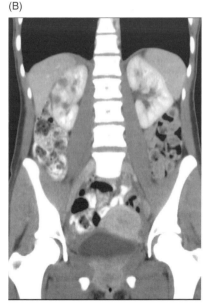

Renal lymphoma before (A) and after (B) treatment. Large hypodense masses expanding the right kidney prior to treatment, with significant reduction in volume of the lesions post-treatment.

Pancreas

- Primary pancreatic lymphoma is responsible for just over 1% of pancreatic neoplasms and is more common in NHL than HD.
- A large pancreatic mass, with only mild pancreatic duct and common bile duct obstruction, associated with retroperitoneal nodal involvement is highly suspicious of lymphoma.

Genitourinary tract

- Although rarely involved in early disease, involvement rises to 50% in advanced lymphoma.
- The testicle is most commonly involved, followed by kidney and perirenal space. Involvement of the prostate, bladder, uterus, vagina and ovaries is documented but rare.
- Testicular lymphoma is the commonest form of testicular neoplasm in patients over 60 years.
- It is found in 1% of men with NHL, almost never in HD. Many cases are clinically silent and the testis is an important site of residual disease following treatment at other sites (similar to CNS disease). US demonstrates non-specific findings of focal areas of hypoechogenicity or diffuse decreased testicular echogenicity. It is bilateral in over 20% of patients.

- Renal involvement is a relatively late event, with disease remaining clinically silent in many patients.
- Renal function usually remains normal and in 90% is caused by high-grade NHL.
- Involvement usually produces multiple intrarenal masses (60%). On CT, these show typical density reversal patterns on both NECT and CECT. In 10–20%, a solitary mass, indistinguishable from carcinoma, is noted.
- Renal involvement occurs in the absence of retroperitoneal adenopathy in over half of those affected. Direct infiltration of the kidneys from the retroperitoneum via the renal hilum is the second commonest mode of involvement.
- A soft tissue mass in the perirenal space is also commonly seen, encasing the kidney without apparently invading it.
- Diffuse renal involvement and subsequent enlargement and patchy non-enhancement are less commonly seen.
- Secondary involvement of the bladder is found in 10–15% of patients: on CT and MRI this appears either as diffuse widespread bladder wall thickening or as a large nodular mass. Both of these are indistinguishable from transitional cell carcinoma and result in haematuria.
- Primary bladder lymphoma is a MALT type and is more common in women with a history of cystitis, presenting as solitary or multiple sessile masses.
- Involvement of the prostate is usually diffuse, with direct extension from pelvic side wall nodes, in advanced disease, being the most common form.
- Female genital tract involvement in advanced lymphoma is common, though primary involvement is rare (1% of extra-nodal NHL).
- Most cases involve postmenopausal women, presenting with postmenopausal bleeding. Lymphoma may affect the cervix or uterine body, where it produces diffuse enlargement with homogeneous signal return or enhancement. Characteristically, the uterine mucosa is uninvolved and the low-signal-intensity junctional zone, seen on MRI, remains intact.
- Ovarian lymphoma is rare but carries a poor prognosis because of the advanced stage of disease at this point. Lesions are characteristically bilateral and show homogeneous enhancement without haemorrhage, necrosis or calcification.

Adrenal glands

- Primary involvement is rare; however in diffuse lymphoma, secondary involvement occurs in 4% as assessed on CT, and in 24% of postmortem examinations.
- Occurs more commonly with NHL than HD.

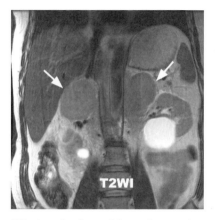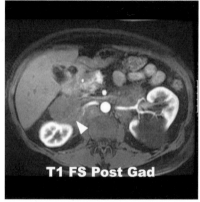

Bilateral adrenal lymphoma in a patient with HIV. The coronal T2W MRI demonstrates large, heterogeneous, faintly hyperintense adrenal masses (arrows). Following the administration of gadolinium (Post Gad), only minimal enhancement is demonstrated (arrowhead).

- Bilateral involvement is seen in 50% of patients.
- Usually characterized as an area of low signal intensity on T1W images and as an area of heterogeneous high signal intensity on T2W images, with minimal progressive enhancement after contrast.

New developments

- The recent introduction of ^{18}F-FDG PET-CT has contributed significantly to the detection and assessment of lymphoma.
- Cross-sectional imaging (CT, MRI and US) depends on the detection of abnormalities in size, appearance and enhancement for the diagnosis of organ involvement in lymphoma.
- Lymphomatous involvement often does not lead to anatomical changes on imaging.
- This is particularly important in the assessment of post-treatment potential residual/recurrent disease. Functional imaging with ^{18}F-FDG PET-CT enables a semiquantitative assessment of functionally abnormal tissue and has become increasingly central to imaging in lymphoma.

Omental secondary deposits

Clinical characteristics

- The omentum is a fold of visceral peritoneum related to the stomach and transverse colon, containing a large amount of fat and a rich vascular network.
- Secondary neoplasms of the omentum are more common than primary neoplasms. Ovarian carcinoma is the most common primary neoplasm metastasising to omentum.
- Spread is either direct along the transverse mesocolon, the gastrosplenic or gastrocolic ligaments or via peritoneal or haematogenous spread.
- The patient may be asymptomatic but there may be indicators of progression of their underlying malignancy, with rising levels of tumour markers.

Radiological features

- Omental deposits are visible on both US and CT. They may be detected earlier on CT as irregular soft tissue density in the omental fat.
- In more advanced disease, the deposits range from discrete nodules to confluent solid masses known as omental cakes. These may enhance. Additional peritoneal deposits may be seen.
- MRI using gadolinium enhancement with fat suppression is also sensitive for omental and peritoneal secondaries; the deposits show as enhancing soft tissue lesions against the background of the dark suppressed fat.

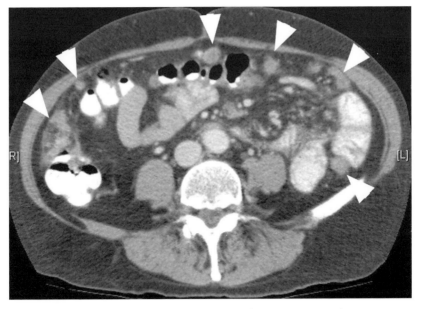

Multiple peritoneal nodules (arrowheads) in a patient with ovarian carcinoma.

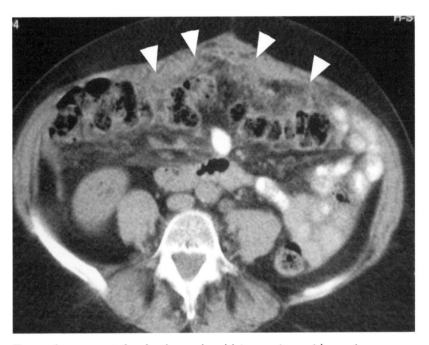

Extensive omental cake (arrowheads) in a patient with ovarian carcinoma.

Pancreatic carcinoma

Clinical characteristics

- Subtypes include carcinoma arising from ductal elements (ductal carcinoma), carcinoma arising from the glandular elements (pancreatic acinar carcinoma), tumours arising from the endocrine component of the pancreas (islet cell cancer, glucagonoma, gastrinoma, VIPoma, somatostatinoma and non-functioning islet cell tumour). Metastases to the pancreas occur but are uncommon.
- This discussion will focus on pancreatic ductal carcinoma.
- Ductal carcinoma accounts for 80–90% of non-endocrine pancreatic cancer and is the fifth leading cause of cancer death in Western countries.
- There is increased risk with alcohol abuse, diabetes, heredity and African ancestry.
- A number of oncogene mutations have been identified including *p53* and k-*ras* mutations, as well as overexpression of growth factors such as epidermal growth factor and transforming growth factor.
- There is an increasing incidence with age, ductal carcinoma being most common in the 7th decade.
- Over 50% of lesions are located in the head, 25% in the body and approximately 10% in the tail.
- Spread is through the pancreas into adjacent structures, with local nodal and subsequent metastases to liver (30%), lungs, pleura and bone. Peritoneal carcinomatosis with ascites occurs in up to 10% of patients.
- Local extension is predominantly posterior, involving visceral vessels and the retroperitoneum. Extension anteriorly or laterally into the splenic hilum also occurs.
- Local extension may result in a tumour mass involving pancreas, duodenum, porta hepatis, spleen, stomach, root of small-bowel mesentery and particularly the left adrenal gland.
- In 85% of patients presenting with ductal adenocarcinoma, there will be extra-pancreatic extension at the time of presentation and the carcinoma is incurable.
- At presentation, 40% have lymph node metastases, 50% have hepatic metastases and 35% have peritoneal implants.
- Median survival is 12–18 months. It has the worst 5-year survival of more than 60 human malignancies.
- Clinical features depend on the extent of disease and the site of origin.
- In general, tumours in the head produce earlier symptoms than more distal tumours, because of early involvement of the common bile duct as it passes through the head of the pancreas to empty into the second part of the duodenum.

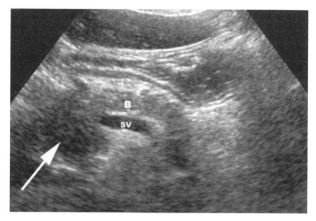

Pancreatic carcinoma. Ill-defined hypoechoic mass within the head of pancreas (arrow) on US. B, body of pancreas; SV, splenic vein.

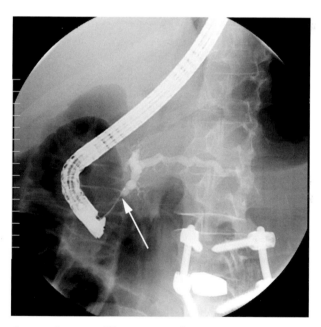

Pancreatic carcinoma. Obstruction of the pancreatic duct owing to a mass within the head of pancreas (arrow) shown on ERCP.

- Signs of head of pancreas lesions include obstructive jaundice. Pancreatic carcinoma is the commonest cause of malignant biliary obstruction (75%).
- In less central lesions, or in advanced local disease, symptoms include severe central back pain (involvement of retroperitoneal nerves), portal

thrombophlebitis and thrombosis (direct extension into vein or para-neoplastic syndrome), diabetes (destruction of islet cells by tumour) and fatigue, malaise and weight loss (pancreatic insufficiency and paraneo-plastic disease).

Radiological features

- The goals of imaging include accurate preoperative staging to identify the small proportion of patients where curative pancreaticoduodenec-tomy may be considered, and to diagnose mimics of ductal adenocarci-noma that have a significantly better prognosis.
- In patients with obvious extra-pancreatic extension (where curative surgery is not possible), CT- or US-guided fine needle aspiration is standard procedure to confirm imaging diagnosis. In small tumours, endoscopic US-guided fine needle aspiration can be used to improve diagnostic yield.
- In general, MRI and CECT are the most widely used modalities for imaging and are roughly equivalent in their accuracy for tumour iden-tification, local staging and identification of distant metastases.
- The role of ^{18}F-FDG PET is evolving and it may become more useful in the differentiation of benign and malignant lesions, and the identifica-tion of distant metastases.
- Pancreatic ductal carcinomas are relatively avascular compared with normal pancreatic tissue, while islet cell tumours are hypervascular. These features are utilised by subsequent imaging techniques.
- Patient preparation for CECT includes distension of stomach and duodenum with 1000 ml of water orally. Initial NECT of target area is followed by a late arterial phase scan. This arterial phase improves visualisation of ductal carcinoma through its relative hypoattenuation, a result of its relatively hypovascular nature, compared with the normal pancreatic tissue.
- This phase also enhances visualisation of small hepatic metastases by showing ring enhancement.
- Islet cell tumours, which are hypervascular, readily show up against pancreatic tissue during arterial phase.
- Venous phase scanning at 70s serves to confirm liver metastases, portal venous occlusion and venous collaterals in portal obstruction.
- Curved planar reconstructions through the pancreas can demonstrate the pancreatic duct, common bile duct and peripancreatic vasculature. Of particular importance is involvement of the superior mesenteric vasculature.
- Arterial encasement by tumour is an absolute contraindication to sur-gical resection.
- Obliteration of fat planes around 50% of the circumference of a vessel on both MRI and CECT is reliable in predicting vascular involvement.

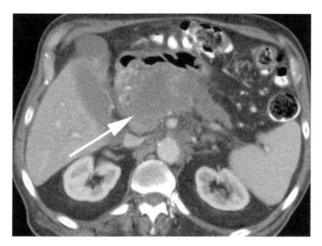

Carcinoma of the head of pancreas. Ill-defined mass replacing the head of pancreas (arrow) seen on CECT, with extension into the adjacent body and invasion of the second part of duodenum.

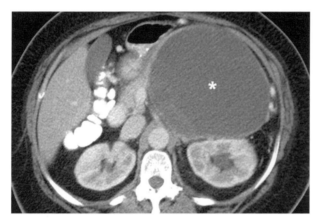

Pancreatic mucinous cystadenocarcinoma. Large, faintly septated, cystic neoplasm (asterisk) effacing the body and tail of pancreas.

- Involvement of the portal venous system is controversial, with some surgeons still opting for attempted curative surgery.
- Most tumours (except uncinate process tumours) lead to eventual involvement and obstruction of the common bile duct. Tumours in the head and uncinate process typically infiltrate along the superior mesenteric artery and root of small-bowel mesentery, while tumours within the tail extend into splenic hilar structures and coeliac and hepatic vessels.
- Direct extension into bowel wall is often visualised as an infiltrating hypovascular mass involving the strongly enhancing bowel wall.

- Assessment of nodal involvement is difficult. Pancreatic carcinoma drains to peripancreatic nodes, then to nodes in the porta hepatis and root of small-bowel mesentery, and finally to peri-aortic and distal superior mesenteric nodes. Nodes >1 cm are considered involved. However, there is a high propensity for micrometastases in pancreatic carcinoma, with no subsequent nodal enlargement. In addition, reactive adenopathy following coexistent pancreatitis or instrumentation (ERCP) is common, and nodal evaluation by CT is poor.
- Metastases to liver and peritoneal surfaces are the most frequently observed intra-abdominal sites. Small hepatic metastases are detected during late arterial enhancement by ring enhancement. Peritoneal thickening, nodules and ascites are indications of peritoneal involvement.
- Fast MR techniques, such as echo planar imaging and three-dimensional volumetric breath holding, have established MR as a CT equivalent tool for initial diagnosis and staging. The most useful sequence is contrast-enhanced T1W breath-hold gradient echo sequences. MRCP is useful for visualising the pancreatic duct or common bile duct obstruction or involvement.
- Pancreatic ductal carcinoma generally has a lower signal intensity than normal pancreatic tissue, particularly with fat-suppression techniques. T2W images are utilised for detection of hepatic metastases, showing little contrast difference within the pancreas itself. Fast spin-echo techniques are utilised for pancreatic visualisation owing to their rapid acquisition and gadolinium-enhanced T1W echo gradient sequences are used to map vascular invasion.
- Endoscopic US plays a useful role in local staging when there is no CECT or MRI evidence of distant metastases. Carcinoma is typically hypoechoic on US and ductal obstruction distal to the lesion is readily visualised on endoscopic US. Where tumour is unresectable, a definitive tissue diagnosis may be obtained by endoscopic US-guided fine needle aspiration.
- Use of ^{18}F-FDG PET is sensitive and specific for pancreatic malignancy, with sensitivity of 88% and specificity of 83%. It is useful in differentiating benign from malignant lesions, confirming possible liver and peritoneal metastases as identified on CECT or MRI, and is useful in the follow-up of patients in the context of a rising carbohydrate antigen 19-9 (CA19-9) serology.
- Upper GI tract contrast studies are currently less utilised for diagnosis and generally are performed in the context of postsurgical or palliative management. However, on occasion, they may be the first indicator of pancreatic malignancy, which may be demonstrated as an irregular or smooth nodular mass, in the case of an ampullary lesion, or spiculation and traction of the duodenum, in the case of local extension from a head or body cancer. Extrinsic indentation of the ampulla of the duodenum may be seen.

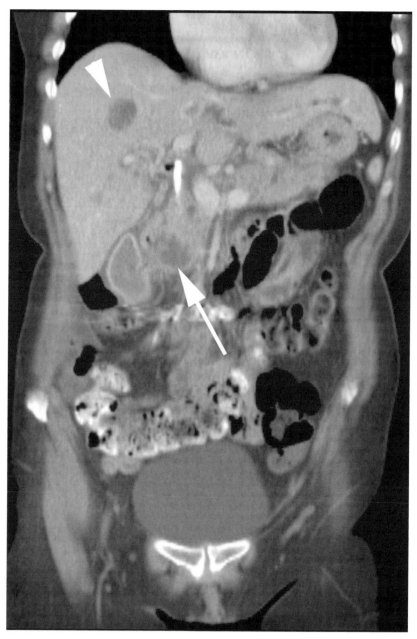

Carcinoma of the head of pancreas. Coronal reformat CECT shows an ill-defined hypodense mass within the head of pancreas (arrow) with a fairly well-defined hypodense metastasis within the right lobe of liver (arrowhead).

Pancreatitis

Clinical characteristics

- Classified as acute and chronic.
- Alcohol and cholelithiasis account for 60–70% of cases.
- Cholelithiasis responsible for 75% of cases of acute pancreatitis.
- Alcohol responsible for 70% of chronic pancreatitis cases.
- In 20–30% less common causes are involved, including metabolic disorders (often with hypercalcaemia and/or hyperlipidaemia as common factors), multiple myeloma, amyloidosis and sarcoidosis.
- Hereditary pancreatitis is an autosomal dominant disorder producing early-onset recurrent pancreatitis, with 20–40% developing pancreatic carcinoma.
- Other causes include trauma, surgery, viral infections, such as measles and mononucleosis, parasites, structural abnormalities, such as pancreas divisum, and drugs such as steroids and thiazide diuretics.
- Up to 20% of cases are idiopathic.
- **Complications** include:
  - pancreatic necrosis.
  - acute peripancreatic fluid collections (phlegmon).
  - pseudocyst formation.
  - pancreatic abscess.

Clinical presentation

- Mild acute pancreatitis presents with epigastric abdominal pain, often radiating through to the back, associated with nausea, vomiting and general malaise.
- Occasionally progresses to acute severe pancreatitis, with profound systemic upset including shock, adult respiratory distress syndrome (ARDS) and multiorgan failure, flank ecchymosis (Grey-Turner sign) and peri-umbilical ecchymosis (Cullen sign).
- Chronic pancreatitis presents with chronic intermittent abdominal pain and symptoms and signs of pancreatic insufficiency, including malabsorption, diabetes mellitus and occasionally obstructive jaundice.
- Patients may also present with complications of acute pancreatitis, such as jaundice from oedema of the common bile duct or calculi, pain and upper GI obstructive symptoms (from pseudocyst formation) and diabetes from islet cell destruction.

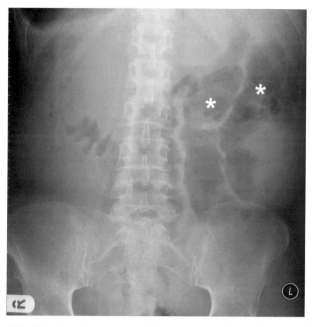

Pancreatitis. Sentinel loops in the left upper quadrant (asterisks) secondary to pancreatitis.

Acute pancreatitis

Radiological features

- **AXR:**
  - 'Sentinel loop' – localised segment of gas-filled small bowel caused by peritonism – is typically seen in the upper abdomen.
  - 'Colon cutoff sign': dilated transverse colon with abrupt change to a gasless descending colon, caused by local inflammation resulting in spasm of the splenic flexure.
  - Mottled appearance of pancreatic region owing to fat necrosis.
  - Gas-less abdomen: multiple loops of fluid-filled bowel.
  - Ascites.
  - Intrapancreatic gas bubbles caused by necrosis and abscess formation.
  - Gallstones may be identified if calcified.
  - None of these findings is specific and usually CT and/or US are more helpful.
- **CXR:**
  - Left-sided pleural effusion.
  - Left-sided hemidiaphragmatic elevation.
  - Left-sided basal atelectasis.

- Pulmonary oedema or infiltrates in ARDS.
- Occasionally a pericardial effusion complicates pancreatitis.
- None of these findings are specific.
- **USS:**
  - Hypoechoic enlarged gland, caused by diffuse oedema.
  - The pancreatic duct may be dilated (not normally seen in the normal gland).
  - Complications of acute pancreatitis (vide infra).
- **Barium meal and follow through:**
  - Enlarged tortuous rugal folds.
  - Widening of retrogastric space (from pancreatic enlargement/inflammation in lesser sac).
  - Diminished duodenal peristalsis from surrounding inflammation.
  - Oedematous swelling of papilla of Vater: Poppel sign.
  - These studies have been largely superseded by CT and US.
- **CECT:**
  - Normal appearance of pancreas in nearly 30%.
  - Enlarged and indistinct gland as a result of oedema.
  - Thickening of anterior pararenal fascia.
  - Hyperdense intrapancreatic portion can represent haemorrhagic pancreatitis.
  - Hypodense intrapancreatic portion may be seen, representing phlegmonous pancreatitis.
  - Non-enhancing areas indicate necrotic pancreatitis.
- **MRI:**
  - Inflammatory change in the peripancreatic fat is well demonstrated on T2W fat-saturated images. Areas of non-enhancement indicate necrosis.
  - MRI is generally used to investigate possible aetiologies, using MRCP to demonstrate gallstones not identified on US or CT.

Chronic pancreatitis

Radiological features

- **AXR:** multiple irregular pancreatic calcifications are virtually pathognomonic. More commonly seen in alcohol-related disease.
- **USS:**
  - Atrophic, bright pancreas, often with focal or extensive irregular duct dilatation.
  - Intraductal calcifications.
  - Less commonly focal or diffuse glandular enlargement, mainly caused by mild biliary duct dilatation.

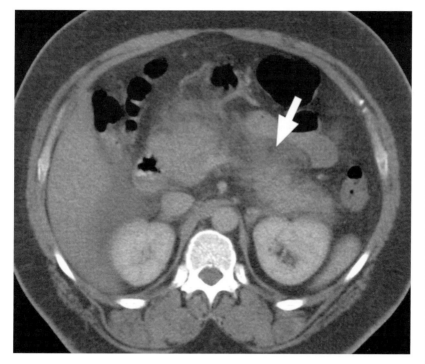

Acute pancreatitis. Swollen enhancing pancreas with extensive peripancreatic inflammatory soft tissue stranding (arrow).

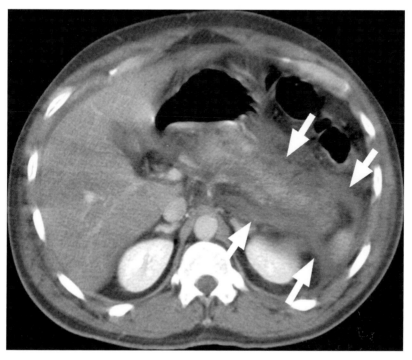

Acute pancreatitis. Diffusely swollen pancreas with extensive peripancreatic inflammatory free fluid (arrows).

- **CT (pre- and postcontrast):**
  - Similar findings to those with US.
  - NECT is excellent for demonstrating minimal degrees of pancreatic calcification.
  - CECT allows further characterisation of necrotic areas or intra/peri-pancreatic fluid collections.
  - Allows assessment of regional damage caused by recurrent inflammation (e.g. damage to the duodenum).
- **MRI:**
  - Loss of signal intensity on T1W fat-suppressed images results from loss of aqueous protein from pancreatic acini owing to fibrosis.
  - Suboptimal contrast enhancement on post-gadolinium T1W images results from destruction of the vascular tree by fibrosis.
- **Cholangiopancreatography:**
  - Increasing use of MRCP has to a degree supplanted the use of ERCP.
  - Key finding is irregular dilatation of pancreatic duct (grade I–III).
  - Ranges from slight duct ectasia to beading of main duct with intra-ductal protein plugs.
  - Filling defects may represent calculi.

Complications of pancreatitis

Pancreatic necrosis

- Release of proteolytic and procoagulant enzymes within the pancreas leads to diffuse necrosis.
- CECT is 90% accurate for diagnosis, demonstrating non-enhancement of necrotic tissue.
- Often associated with other complications, for example ARDS, widespread fat necrosis.
- Prognosis depends on degree of necrosis, rising to 50% mortality with 90% glandular necrosis.

Infected pancreatic necrosis

- Necrotic pancreatic tissue that becomes infected.
- May occur at any time following pancreatitis.
- CECT: gas-forming organisms produce pockets of gas within non-enhancing necrotic pancreatic tissue.
- Open surgical debridement and drainage required.
- Prognosis worse than for pancreatic abscess.

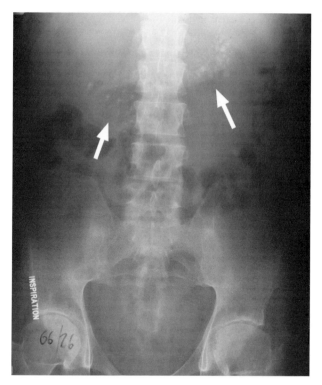

Chronic pancreatitis. Secondary multifocal coarse pancreatic calcification (arrows).

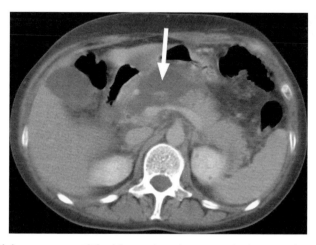

Necrotising pancreatitis. Non-enhancing necrotic tissue within the head and proximal body of the pancreas (arrow).

Acute fluid collections (phlegmon)

- Collections of *enzyme-rich* fluid anterior to pancreas.
- Occurs in ~40% of patients with acute pancreatitis.
- Usually anterior and peripheral to gland.
- No fibrous capsule, as opposed to pseudocyst formation.
- Because of the proteolytic nature of the fluid, the collection can readily spread into the mediastinum, pararenal fascia and neighbouring organs (e.g. liver and spleen).
- Resolution is spontaneous in 50% and only requires serial follow-up.
- In the other 50% pseudocysts develop or complications of superadded infection or haemorrhage occur.
- Often only distinguishing factor from pseudocyst is resolution on serial imaging.
- On CECT, the collection presents as a hypodense area of water density (<10HU) within the pancreatic bed, which may persist for months.

Pancreatic pseudocyst

- A collection of pancreatic fluid that is encysted in a fibrous wall.
- Occurs approximately 1 month after the acute onset of pancreatitis.
- Usually oval or round in configuration.
- Two-thirds are located within the pancreas itself but can occasionally be intraperitoneal, retroperitoneal, intraparenchymal or mediastinal.
- Caused by microperforation of the pancreatic duct, leading to an encapsulated collection of fluid and enzymes.
- Follows acute pancreatitis in up to 10% of patients. May also been seen in those with chronic pancreatitis.
- Usually sterile but may become secondarily infected, leading to abscess formation.
- Of pseudocysts, 50% resolve spontaneously and pose no problems, 20% are stable and 30% lead to complications including:
  - severe haemorrhage caused by erosion into superior mesenteric vessels.
  - splenic vein thrombosis from adjacent inflammation and pressure.
  - peritonitis caused by rupture into the peritoneal cavity, lesser or greater sac.
  - dissection into adjacent organs such as liver, spleen or posterior wall of stomach.
  - pressure obstruction of duodenum or common bile duct, leading to jaundice and cholangitis.
  - superadded infection.
  - increasing size through communication with pancreatic duct or haemorrhage and osmosis.

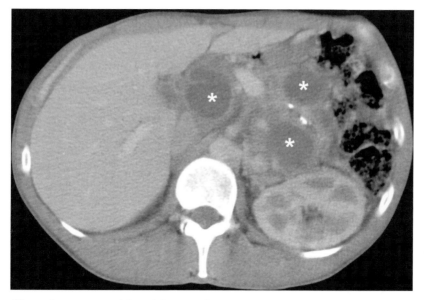

Chronic pancreatitis with pseudocyst formation. Multiple peripancreatic pseudocysts (asterisks). Note the pancreatic calcification typical of chronic pancreatitis.

- **AXR:**
  - Indentation of posterior stomach wall by cyst.
  - Indirect evidence of pancreatic mass (e.g. displacement of the splenic flexure, downward displacement of duodenojejunal junction.
  - Gastric outlet obstruction.
  - Not sensitive or specific.
- **USS:**
  - Usually a unilocular single hypoechoic cyst is seen in relation to pancreas.
  - Multilocular in under 10%.
  - May contain internal echoes owing to debris, haemorrhage, cellular debris.
- **CECT:** fluid-filled peripancreatic cyst of 0–30 HU attenuation.
- **ERCP:** communication with pancreatic duct in 70%.

Pancreatic abscess

- Fluid collection, often in relation to the pancreas, containing bacteria and pus.
- Usually occurs 4 weeks after acute pancreatitis.
- Enhancement of abscess capsule on CECT.
- Managed by percutaneous drainage.

Portal vein thrombosis

- In the majority of cases, no cause for portal vein thrombosis is evident, in spite of extensive investigation.
- More common in children and young adults.
- Secondary causes include:
  - trauma: accidental, intraoperative or following umbilical vein cannulation.
  - tumour invasion, typically in hepatocellular carcinoma, cholangio-carcinoma and pancreatic carcinoma.
  - blood dyscrasias leading to hypercoagulable states, such as sickle cell disease and severe dehydration (again more common in children).
  - intra-abdominal sepsis.
  - cirrhosis and portal hypertension, presumably owing to altered hae-modynamics and venous stasis.
- May be isolated with relatively few effects or may result in:
  - portal hypertension, with its associated complications.
  - extension of thrombosis into mesenteric vessels, with subsequent small-bowel infarction.
  - hepatic infarction: two-thirds of the hepatic blood flow is derived from the portal vein.

Clinical characteristics

- Most commonly seen in children.
- Hepatic encephalopathy as a result of diversion of portal blood through the systemic circulation.
- Abdominal pain.
- Haematemesis secondary to oesophageal varices.

Radiological features

- **AXR:**
  - Shows hepatosplenomegaly.
  - Not very sensitive.

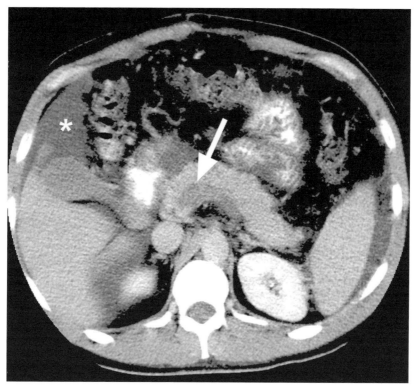

Portal vein thrombosis. Non-opacification of the porto-splenic venous confluence (arrow) and distal splenic vein. Note the presence of ascites (asterisk).

- **USS:**
  - Best imaging modality for screening in high-risk cases (lack of radiation is especially useful in the younger target age group).
  - Portal thrombosis appears as intraluminal material, of variable echogenicity, in an enlarged portal vein.
  - Presence of portal hypertension can be confirmed by direct Doppler interrogation of the portal vein and presence of porto-systemic collaterals and ascites.
  - Decrease in hepatic arterial resistive index – a value of <0.5 is highly suggestive – as a result of a partial compensatory increase in arterial flow. This may be helpful in differentiating acute from chronic portal vein thrombosis, as a fall in the index is not seen in the chronic condition or in non-occlusive thrombosis (e.g. malignant thrombus).
  - Cavernous transformation may be evident in subacute or chronic thrombosis: a thrombosed extrahepatic portal vein is seen, with multiple cavernous channels at the porta hepatis.
- **CT:** typical appearances of intraluminal thrombosis:
  - hyperdense thrombus on non-enhancing CT.
  - hypodense filling defect surrounded by contrast on CECT.
- **MRI:**
  - Collaterals appear as multiple tubular flow voids.
  - Portal vein thrombus is bright on T1W images.
- **Angiography:**
  - Thrombus appears as a filling defect on mesenteric venography.
  - Tumour thrombus may appear as streaky contrast-filled vessels within the thrombus-filling defect.

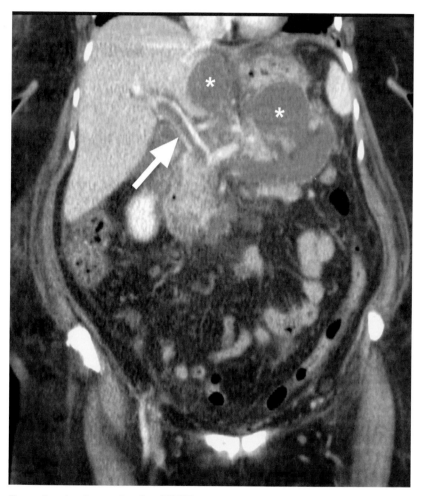

Portal vein thrombosis. CECT coronal reformat shows filling defect
within the portal vein, representing thrombus (arrow), secondary to
pancreatitis. Note the large secondary hypodense pseudocysts (asterisks).

Portal venous gas

- Bacterial overgrowth and invasion of the colonic submucosal venous plexus can lead to gas in the portal system. This results in portal venous flow carrying gas to the liver.
- In the adult, it is usually a result of bowel wall infarction and impending gangrene, and carries a very poor prognosis. Often a pre-terminal event.
- The aetiology usually involves intestinal necrosis from a variety of causes. The most common include:
  - arterial or venous occlusion leading to bowel infarction.
  - any severe inflammatory colonic condition such as severe UC, severe diverticular disease or intra-abdominal abscess.
  - severe necrotising pancreatitis can also result in portal gas from subsequent adjacent colonic inflammation.
  - necrotising enterocolitis.
  - perforated peptic ulceration.
- In children, often accompanies bowel obstruction, most commonly from some form of congenital atresia such as oesophageal or duodenal atresia.
- Also seen in relation to umbilical vein catheterisation in sick neonates.
- A relatively common finding in neonatal necrotising enterocolitis, where, in contrast to adults, it does not carry the same poor prognosis.
- Other, less-common, causes include iatrogenic injection of gas during colonoscopy, air embolism during barium enema procedures, pneumonia and diabetes.

Clinical characteristics

- There are no distinct clinical features.
- Often just part of the picture in a severely ill adult or neonate.
- Its significance is as an indicator of severe sepsis or bowel infarction.
- It is a worse prognostic sign in adults than in neonates.

Radiological features

- **AXR:**
  - Often a subtle finding, which may be transient, especially in neonates with necrotising enterocolitis.
  - Typically presents as peripheral hepatic branching linear lucencies.
  - Gas may occasionally be seen in the intestinal wall (pneumatosis intestinalis) and less commonly in the mesenteric vessels themselves.

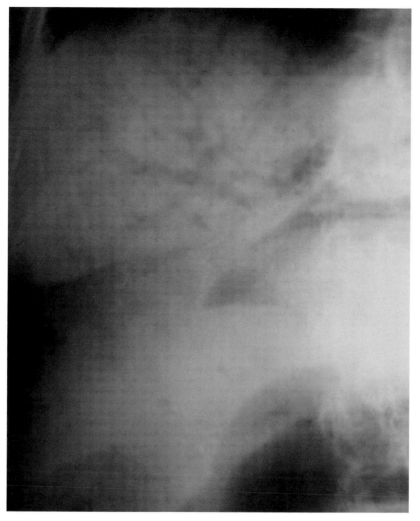

Portal venous gas caused by bowel necrosis. Note the branching lucencies within the portal venules, extending peripherally to the liver edge.

- **USS:**
  - Gas in the portal venules within the liver produces intensely echogenic foci, often described as a 'snow storm' appearance.
  - Doppler US reveals sharp bidirectional spikes superimposed on the normal portal vein signal, caused by almost total reflection of sound waves from microscopic portal gas bubbles.
- **CT:**
  - Both NECT and CECT are exceptionally sensitive to the presence of air.
  - Portal vein gas is often difficult to distinguish from pneumobilia. In gas within the intrahepatic bile ducts, the gas is often seen in a more central position within the liver. This is presumably because of the central flow direction of bile, carrying gas bubbles towards the porta hepatis, whereas the portal flow carries the gas towards the periphery of the liver.

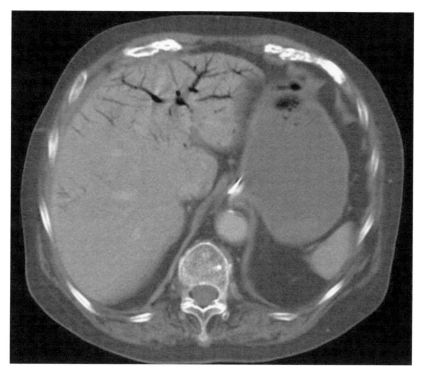

Portal venous gas. Extensive gas seen predominantly within the left lobe of liver, secondary to bowel necrosis.

Portal venous hypertension

- Defined as a portal venous pressure of more than 5–10mmHg.
- Almost always caused by increased portal venous resistance.
- Site of resistance may be pre-, intra- or post-hepatic.
- *Prehepatic* causes include portal venous thrombosis and portal venous compression from tumour, lymphadenopathy or pancreatic masses including a pseudocyst.
- *Intrahepatic* causes include obstruction at the pre-sinusoidal, sinusoidal and post-sinusoidal levels:
  - pre-sinusoidal: congenital hepatic fibrosis, idiopathic non-cirrhotic fibrosis, primary biliary cirrhosis.
  - sinusoidal: hepatitis, sickle cell disease.
  - post-sinusoidal: cirrhosis and veno–occlusive hepatic disease.
- *Post-hepatic* causes are increased resistance to hepatic venous outflow, as in congestive heart failure, constrictive pericarditis and Budd–Chiari syndrome.
- The most common cause world wide is schistosomiasis. In Western countries, it is probably alcohol-induced cirrhosis, followed by hepatitis C-induced cirrhosis.
- Less-common causes include hyperdynamic flow states through the portal venous system. These are mainly caused by abnormal vascular channels in either hepatocellular carcinoma, or congenital arteriovenous fistulae in conditions such as Osler–Weber–Rendu syndrome or traumatic arteriovenous fistula formation.
- Whatever the underlying aetiology, elevated portal venous pressure leads to diversion of GI venous return from the portal system to the systemic circulation via *porto-systemic collateral vessels*.
- Porto-systemic collateral vessels include:
  - Coronary vein to azygos or hemi-azygos system via lower oesophageal veins.
  - Superior and inferior mesenteric veins to iliac veins via mesenteric varices.
  - Para-umbilical and omental veins to superficial veins of chest and anterior abdominal wall via *caput medusae* veins.
  - Splenic vein to azygos system via gastric fundal veins in gastrosplenic ligament, producing splenic hilar varices.
  - Gastric veins to renal veins via gastro–renal anastomoses.
  - Gastric veins to pulmonary veins via gastric and pericardiophrenic collaterals.
  - Inferior mesenteric veins to internal iliac veins via rectal haemorrhoidal veins.

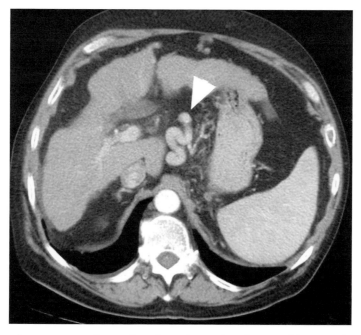

Large lower oesophageal varices (arrowhead) caused by portal hypertension. Note the irregular outline of the liver owing to chronic liver disease.

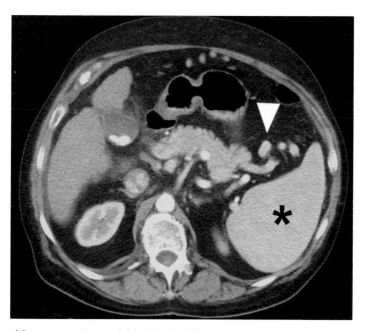

Portal hypertension with splenic hilar varices (arrowhead; same patient as above). Evidence of chronic liver disease and splenomegaly (asterisk). Gallstones in gallbladder.

- Splenic veins to retroperitoneal venous system via duodenal and retroperitoneal varices.
  - Intrahepatic shunt from portal to hepatic veins.
- Portal venous congestion also produces splenomegaly, ascites and GI congestion.

Clinical characteristics

- Dilated porto-systemic collaterals (varices), particularly in the lower oesophagus and lower rectum, are submucosal in position, structurally weak and easily traumatised, and may undergo torrential haemorrhage.
- Drainage of blood from the GI system, directly into the systemic venous circulation, bypasses the detoxifying function of the liver and may lead to hepatic encephalopathy.
- Increased portal pressure produces local GI mucosal congestion, leading to GI bleeding, malabsorption, splenomegaly and ascites.
- Underlying liver damage potentiates the effects of malabsorption and haemorrhage.

Radiological features

- **USS:**
  - Enlarged portal vein (abnormal >13 mm diameter).
  - Enlarged superior mesenteric and splenic veins (less useful).
  - Presence of ascites, splenomegaly, evidence of liver disease such as cirrhosis or fibrosis.
  - Presence of porto-systemic collaterals, especially at the splenic hilum, falciform ligament, ligamentum teres of liver (recanalised para-umbilical veins) and lower gasto-oesophageal varices.
  - Important to identify patency of portal and splenic veins as this will influence management.
  - Increased echogenicity and thickening of intrahepatic portal veins.
  - Loss of the normal portal venous pressure fluctuation with respiration; normally portal velocity will increase in expiration.
  - Reduction in portal venous velocity, normally 12–30 cm s^{-1}.
  - Reversal of the normal portal venous flow towards the liver (i.e. hepatofugal flow).
  - Portal hypertension results in an absolute increase in hepatic arterial flow to the liver. This manifests as a dilated hepatic artery with an elevated resistive index, >0.78.
- **Angiography:**
  - Elevated portal pressures (hepatic wedge pressure minus IVC pressure): normal is <5 mmHg.
  - Portal flow towards the liver and porto-systemic collaterals as seen with US.
  - Corkscrew hepatic arteries are fairly indicative.

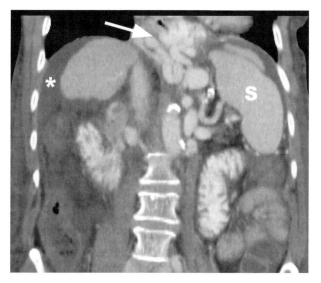

Portal hypertension. CECT (coronal reformat) shows multiple large lower oesophageal varices (arrow), splenomegaly (S), irregular liver edge and ascites (asterisk).

- **CT and MRI:**
  - The presence of ascites, splenomegaly, collateral flow and varices can all be identified on CECT and MRI if disease is advanced enough.
  - Often the underlying liver damage (e.g. cirrhosis or fibrosis) is also evident.

Radiological management

- The most serious complications are hepatic encephalopathy and massive GI haemorrhage from bleeding porto-systemic varices.
- Management is directed towards halting bleeding and reducing portal hypertension.
- **Transjugular intrahepatic porto-systemic shunt (TIPS):**
  - An intrahepatic porto-sytemic shunt to reduce the portal hypertension is formed under radiological control. The procedure involves:
    - percutaneous approach via right internal jugular vein.
    - insertion of an expandable metallic stent between the hepatic and portal veins within the liver substance.
  - Shunt surveillance is with US at regular intervals of 3–6 months.
  - The shunt and collateral morphology, as well as haemodynamics, are assessed at each US assessment.
  - TIPS is a valuable management tool especially in patients with upper GI variceal haemorrhage or refractory ascites and hepatorenal syndrome.
- Complications of TIPS include shunt obstruction, dislodgement and hepatic vein stenosis.
- Operative complications include vascular injury, particularly to the hepatic artery, subcapsular haematoma or intraperitoneal haemorrhage and bile duct damage.
- Although the procedure can lessen portal hypertension, it can worsen hepatic encephalopathy as it will bypass the detoxifying effect of the liver.

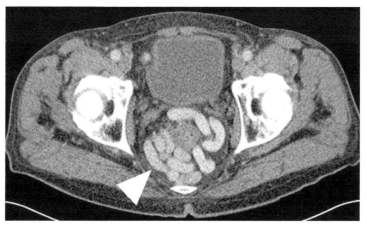

Massive rectal varices secondary to chronic portal venous thrombosis (arrowhead).

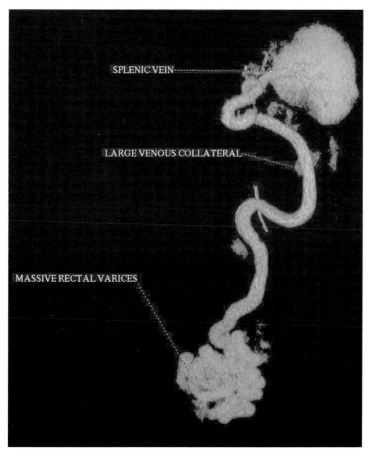

Portal venous thrombosis. Volume rendered image of huge portosystemic collateral circulation, in a patient with chronic portal venous thrombosis.

Pyelonephritis

- Consists of upper urinary tract infection with concomitant pelvicalyceal and parenchymal inflammation.
- Subtypes include emphysematous pyelonephritis, tuberculous pyelonephritis and xanthogranulomatous pyelonephritis.
- Cause is infected urine from lower tract in 80% of adult cases.
- An underlying anatomical abnormality is responsible for 5%:
  - obstruction.
  - ureteric or renal calculus.
  - urinary stasis or reflux.
- Produces wedges of infection extending from papillary tip to cortical surface in patchy distribution, sharply demarcated from adjacent spared parenchyma.
- *Escherichia coli* and *Proteus, Klebsiella, Enterobacter* and *Pseudomonas* spp. responsible for most infections.
- Haematogenous spread with Gram-positive cocci cause 20%.
- Far more common in women, probably because they have shorter urethrae.
- Risk factors include:
  - urinary obstruction (e.g. prostatic hypertrophy in adults).
  - pelviureteric junction obstruction and posterior urethral valve syndrome in children.
  - calculi in any age group.
  - vesicoureteric reflux in children.
  - pregnancy, through hormonal relaxation of ureteral smooth muscle and pressure effects on the ureters.
  - diabetes mellitus.
  - instrumentation of urinary tract.
  - immunosuppression.
  - possibly environmental factors such as dehydration.
- Medical treatment is usually initiated without any imaging.
- Indication for imaging in acute situation:
  - diabetes mellitus.
  - history of renal calculi.
  - underlying renal tract abnormality: anatomical (e.g. scarred kidneys) or functional (e.g. outflow obstruction).
  - growth of atypical organisms.
  - poor clinical response to appropriate antibiotic treatment.
  - frequent recurrences.
  - more than one confirmed episode in a male.
- Management is aimed towards rapid elimination of infecting organism with use of antibiotics and fluid replacement.

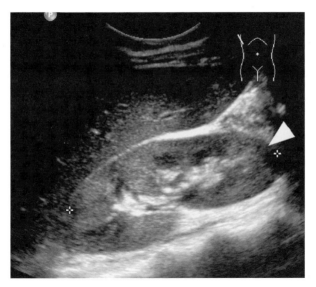

Right pyelonephritis. Large focal area of reduced echogenicity (arrow) replacing the lower half of the right kidney.

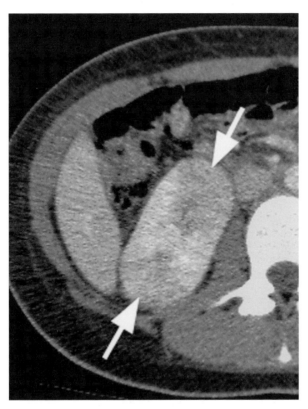

Right pyelonephritis. 'Striated nephrogram' showing stellate hypoattenuating areas from hypoperfusion and oedema.

- In the case of obstruction, this must be relieved as a matter of urgency in the presence of infection, if scarring is to be prevented. This may involve placement of percutaneous nephrostomy or surgical removal of calculi.
- Underlying contributing factors must be dealt with, for example benign prostatic hypertrophy causing outflow obstruction or calculi.
- Medical contributing factors must be controlled (e.g. optimum blood glucose control maintained).

Clinical characteristics

- Presents acutely with signs of generalised sepsis such as fever, chills, leukocytosis.
- Signs of localised infection: flank pain, pyuria and sometimes haematuria, typically microscopic.

Radiological features

- Imaging is important to ensure resolution of acute changes and to exclude anatomical predisposing factors. It is useful in:
  - defining underlying contributing factors such as obstruction, calculi, reflux and previous renal scarring.
  - diagnosing complications including renal and perirenal abscesses and emphysematous pyelonephritis.
  - diagnosing late sequelae, for example scarring, reflux and obstruction.
- **Intravenous urogram:**
  - Renal tract stones ± obstruction may be identified.
  - Normal in over 75% of those with acute uncomplicated pyelonephritis.
  - Renal enlargement may be seen, but this is poorly sensitive.
  - Immediate persistent dense nephrogram is seen, which may be striated.
  - Shows delayed opacification of a collecting system.
  - Compression of collecting system occurs from pyramidal oedema.
  - In severe disease, the kidney cannot be visualised: the aetiology is multifactorial, including interstitial oedema, inflammation, vasculitis and nephron function disruption.
- **USS:**
- Usually normal.
- When abnormal, most common findings are calculi and evidence of obstruction:
  - enlarged kidney(s)
  - decreased echogenicity: either focal or global.
  - loss of central sinus echogenicity owing to fat infiltrated with inflammatory oedema.
  - loss of corticomedullary differentiation.
  - mild hydronephrosis and ureteral dilatation.
  - perirenal fluid from localised perinephric exudates.
  - abscesses or collections.

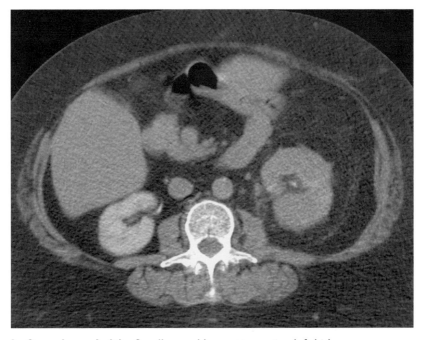

Left pyelonephritis. Swollen and hypoattenuating left kidney.

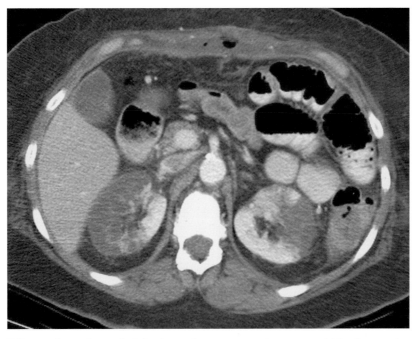

Bilateral pyelonephritis. Large hypoattenuating areas within the renal cortices caused by hypoperfusion and oedema.

- **CT:**
  - Often normal.
  - Localised or generalised renal enlargement identified.
  - Wedge areas of hypoattenuating cortex in early contrast phase owing to hypoperfusion and oedema.
  - Poor corticomedullary differentiation.
  - Mild pelvicalyceal and ureteral dilatation.
  - Thickening of Gerota's fascia.
  - Perirenal stranding, implying perirenal inflammatory changes.
  - Persistent enhancement on delayed scans in areas of diminished enhancement on early phase.
  - Calculi may be seen, as may obstruction.
- **MRI:** wedge-shaped areas of high signal on T1W post-gadolinium sequences.
- **Renal cortical scintigraphy:**
  - Generalised or focal decreased uptake of tracer (usually ^{99m}Tc-labelled DMSA).
  - Reflects decreased nephron function.

Complications of pyelonephritis

Abscesses

- **Renal tract abscesses:**
  - Usually caused by *E. coli* or *Proteus* spp.
  - Cause is an ascending infection in 80%.
  - Cause is haematogenous in 20%; there is a relatively high incidence in IV drug users, endocarditis, blood sepsis and diabetics.
- **Renal abscess:**
  - **IVU:** Focal mass displacing collecting system.
  - **CECT:** non-enhancing low-attenuation intrarenal lesion with enhancing capsule.
  - Gas bubbles may be present and are pathognomonic but not invariable.
  - Perinephric fat obliteration.
  - **USS:** hypoechoic mass with a thickened wall and septations.
  - **NM:** Localised hot spot on galium-67 imaging.
- **Perinephric abscess:**
  - Caused by extension of a renal abscess through the renal capsule.
  - High incidence in diabetics.
  - **CT:** Focal renal mass extending through capsule on cross-sectional imaging.
  - Occasionally gas in renal fossa.
  - **AXR:** shows loss of psoas muscle margin with ipsilateral scoliosis caused by localised muscle spasm, concave towards involved side.

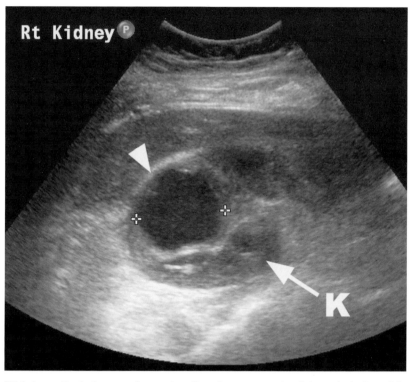

Thick-walled abscess (arrowhead) at the upper pole of the right kidney (K).

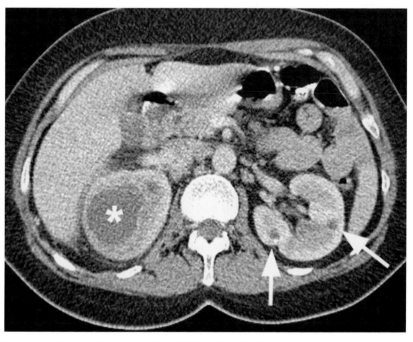

Large right renal abscess (asterisk) and smaller left renal abscesses (arrows).

Xanthogranulomatous pyelonephritis

- Chronic suppurative granulomatous infection in patients with chronic obstruction.
- Usually patients have underlying diabetes mellitus.
- Characterised by parenchymal destruction and replacement with lipid-laden macrophages.
- There is diffuse renal involvement in 90%, with 10% being localised.
- Females are more affected than males; 10% seen in diabetics.
- Large or staghorn calculus seen in 75%, but in 25% is caused by non-calculus obstruction.
- Produces an enlarged non-functioning kidney.
- **USS** may show dilated calyces, low-echo masses, with internal echoes replacing the renal parenchyma.
- **CECT:** the kidney is replaced by multiple non-enhancing low-attenuation masses. The attenuation value of these masses varies from −10 to 30 HU, depending on the lipid content. Caluli are readily apparent.

Emphysematous pyelonephritis

- Usually caused by Gram-negative infection in diabetics.
- Ranges from gas in collecting system alone (emphysematous pyelitis), with a mortality of 20%, to gas in the renal parenchyma and collecting system (emphysematous pyelonephritis), with a mortality of up to 80%.
- **CT:** most reliable in these cases and can detect small pockets of air within the kidney, often extending beyond the capsule and into the renal vein and retroperitoneum.
- **USS:**
  - May demonstrate echogenic foci within the renal parenchyma and sinus caused by gas. Occasionally gas in the perinephric space can obscure the kidney.
  - Treatment is with nephrectomy.

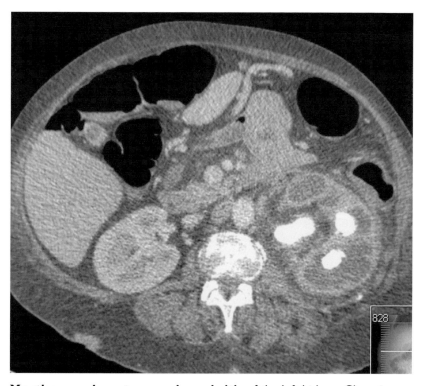

Xanthogranulomatous pyelonephritis of the left kidney. Chronic obstructing calculi and several large non-enhancing masses are seen expanding the left kidney.

Renal artery stenosis

Clinical characteristics

- Renal artery stenosis (RAS) is responsible for up to 4% of cases of hypertension, rising to one in four patients with resistant hypertension and half of those with malignant hypertension.
- Approximately 80% is caused by atherosclerosis; 90% of atherosclerotic stenoses are in the renal artery trunk, usually within 2 cm of its origin.
- The majority of the remainder results from fibromuscular hyperplasia. This is the most common cause of elevated blood pressure in children and young adults and can result in renal insufficiency. This can lead to beading of the artery through alternating stenoses and aneurysmal dilatations. It may also cause a smooth, tubular narrowing. These findings can be subtle.
- Rarer causes include dissection, vasculitis, thromboembolic events and retroperitoneal fibrosis.
- Screening for RAS should be considered in:
  - severe hypertension in young patients.
  - a unilateral atrophic kidney.
  - worsening of renal function following use of an angiotensin-converting enzyme (ACE) inhibitor.
  - hypertension with associated renal impairment of unknown aetiology.
  - long-standing hypertension that rapidly deteriorates.
  - refractory hypertension.
  - presence of abdominal bruit and renal impairment and/or hypertension.
  - vasculopathies with renal impairment and/or hypertension.

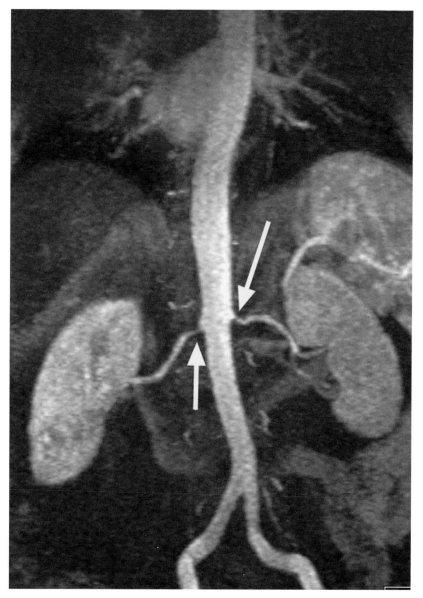

Renal artery stenosis. MR angiography demonstrates bilateral renal artery stenoses (arrows).

Radiological features

- **USS:**
  - A useful imaging technique in assessing renal impairment and hypertension as it can assess renal size, hydronephrosis, renal scarring and masses. It is relatively insensitive for detecting RAS as visualising the renal artery can be difficult in many patients. A further complicating factor is the common occurrence of multiple renal arteries.
  - US usually only helpful in children, very thin adults and in assessing transplant arteries (which are more accessible at US than native arteries).
  - US signs of RAS are:
    - direct visualisation of the stenosis.
    - a peak systolic velocity of $>150\,\mathrm{cm\,s^{-1}}$ with a doppler angle of $<60°$.
    - peak renal artery velocity : peak aortic velocity >3.5.
    - absent diastolic forward flow.
    - spectral broadening, owing to turbulence.
    - dampened waveforms: slow upstroke (*pulsus tardus*) and decreased amplitude (*pulsus parvus*).
- **CECT:**
  - CT angiography using multislice scanners, fine collimation and arterial phase IV enhancement can accurately delineate RAS, but at a high radiation dose.
  - Note that iodinated contrast is nephrotoxic and may cause deterioration in the renal function. Patients should be well hydrated.
- **MR angiography:**
  - Now the first choice for assessing for RAS, with sensitivities of $>95\%$ and specificities of $>90\%$.
  - Although phase contrast and time of flight studies have been used in the past, generally gadolinium-enhanced MR angiography is now used.
  - Can be limited by the presence of a metallic stent. May have difficulty assessing small arteries, either accessory vessels or more distal branches.

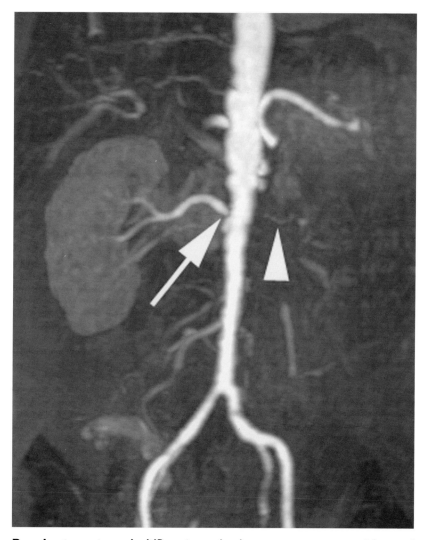

Renal artery stenosis. MR angiography demonstrates a severe right renal artery stenosis (arrow). Note the markedly atrophic left renal artery (arrowhead). See interventional digital subtraction images below.

- **Conventional angiography:**
  - This allows direct visualisation of a RAS.
  - Also allows pressure studies, which help to assess subtle stenosis.
  - Percutaneous transluminal angioplasty and endovascular stent placement are the first-line treatments for RAS.
  - Complications of renovascular intervention include partial or total arterial occlusion owing to thrombosis or dissection, with possible consequent renal infarction. Renal artery spasm can also occur.

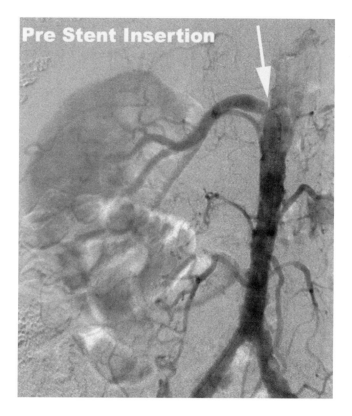

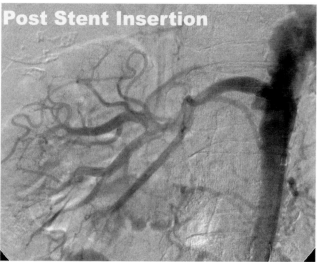

Renal artery digital subtraction angiography. Following the renal MRA (MR angiography (above)), the patient underwent formal renal artery digital subtraction angiography. This confirmed the severe right renal artery stenosis (arrow) and atrophic left renal artery. This was treated with balloon angioplasty and stent insertion, with an excellent end result.

Renal calcification

- Calcification of the renal system may be partial, total, regional, unilateral or bilateral. It may involve just the kidney, part of the organ, or it may be widespread and involve the associated ureter, bladder and seminal vesicles in the male. The causes of calcification are varied but may be classified according to the pattern of involvement.
- Renal calculi are dealt with in a separate section.
- Calcification caused by regional/local disease may involve either part of the kidney or the retroperitoneum.

Perirenal retroperitoneal calcification

- This is usually caused by trauma, infection or neoplasm.
- Traumatic retroperitoneal haematomas often resorb only partially, leaving an area of dystrophic calcification behind.
- The most common neoplasms associated with retroperitoneal calcification are Wilm's tumour, neuroblastoma, teratomas and cavernous haemangioma.
  - Wilms' tumour is the most common solid renal tumour of childhood and may be bilateral in 10%, arising from nephroblastomatosis. The tumour is usually large at presentation, arising from the renal cortex and associated with calcification in about 15%.
  - Neuroblastoma is the most common abdominal malignancy in infancy (cf. Wilms' tumour, which is more common in childhood). It arises from neural crest tissue and presents as a large solid mass, often extending across the midline, encasing the aorta and IVC. It typically produces fine amorphous or stippled calcification (in 85%).
  - Teratomas may occasionally extend to the level of the kidneys. They characteristically produce distinctive calcified structures such as teeth, cartilage and even digits. The appearance is radiologically characteristic.
  - Cavernous haemangiomas of the retroperitoneum demonstrate characteristic calcified phleboliths within their capacious sinusoidal network.

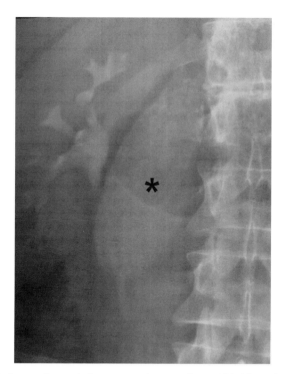

Calcified tuberculous right psoas abscess (asterisk). Note the expansion and bowing of the psoas outline, with lateral displacement of the right kidney.

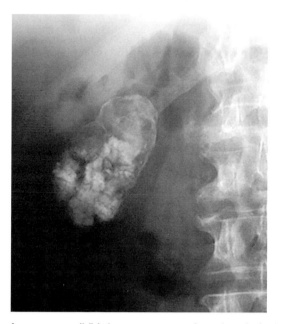

TB autonephrectomy. IVU demonstrates a densely calcified, non-enhancing, small right kidney. The appearances are characteristic of long-standing renal tuberculosis.

Calcification associated with a distinct renal mass

- The differential lies between a renal tumour, cyst, infection or vascular calcification.
- A calcified renal mass should always be investigated further as it may be malignant in up to 75% of cases. The pattern of calcification is also important. Peripheral calcification is usually non-malignant (20%) and is usually calcification in a renal cyst. Non-peripheral calcification is malignant in nearly 90% of occurrences.
- Renal tumours associated with calcification are Wilms' tumour in childhood and renal cell carcinoma in adulthood, where the calcification is often non-peripheral.
- Renal infection with TB often results in calcification of the resulting abscess (*see Tuberculosis*). Characteristic calcifications in a lobar distribution are often seen in end-stage TB: *TB autonephrectomy*.
- Pyogenic abscesses rarely calcify.
- Hydatid disease affects the kidneys in under 5% of patients, but when present calcifies in over 50%.
- Renal cysts demonstrate a spectrum of calcification. Simple cysts very rarely calcify (1%) but intracystic infection or haemorrhage often results in areas of intracystic calcification. In multiple renal cysts, as in adult polycystic disease, peripheral egg-shell calcification is common and much of the kidney becomes replaced by multiple areas of thin egg-shell calcification.
- Vascular calcification associated with a mass may result from either RAS or a renal artery aneurysm, in which case a soft tissue mass is associated with curvilinear or circular egg-shell calcification.

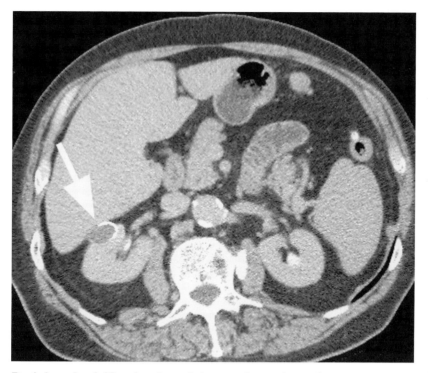

Peripheral calcification in a right renal cyst (arrow).

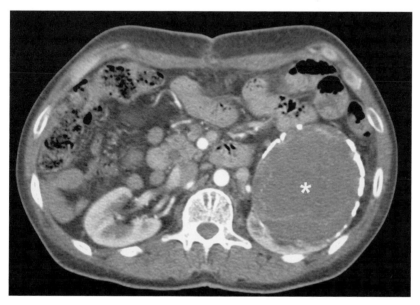

Hydatid disease of the left kidney. A large peripherally calcified cyst (asterisk), containing internal septations, is seen expanding the left kidney.

Nephrocalcinosis

- This is renal parenchymal calcification, which may be cortical or medullary in distribution. Overall incidence varies from under 1% to around 5% of the population and it has a wide spectrum of causes: 95% is medullary nephrocalcinosis with 5% presenting as cortical nephrocalcinosis.

Cortical nephrocalcinosis

- This presents as peripheral (cortical) calcification with sparing of both the subcortical renal region and the medullary pyramids, producing classical 'tramline' calcifications.
- On US the involved kidney demonstrates a highly echogenic cortex.
- The most common causes include:
  - chronic glomerulonephritis.
  - cortical necrosis, most commonly from pregnancy, renovascular shock, infection and renal toxins such as ethylene glycol ingestion (antifreeze).
  - less common causes include Alport's syndrome (hereditary nephritis and deafness), rejected renal transplant and chronic hypercalcaemic states (congenital, paraneoplastic).

Medullary nephrocalcinosis

- In medullary nephrocalcinosis, calcifications involve the distal convoluted tubules within the renal medullary regions.
- **AXR:** There is stippled calcifications of the medullary pyramids.
- **USS:** There is corresponding hyperechogenicity of the involved renal pyramids. The earliest sign may be absence of the relatively hypoechoic renal medulla.
- The most common causes include:
  - hyperparathyroid states, producing chronic hypercalcaemia and hypercalciuria.
  - papillary necrosis (diabetes, cirrhosis, chronic renal obstruction, analgesic abuse and sickle cell disease).
  - medullary sponge kidney.
  - chronic pyelonephritis.
  - other causes of hypercalciuria such as milk alkali syndrome, hypervitaminosis D, renal tubular acidosis, hyperthyroidism, Cushing's syndrome, diabetes mellitus and paraneoplastic syndrome.
  - causes of hyperoxaluria such as hereditary hyperoxaluria and derangements of bile acid metabolism.

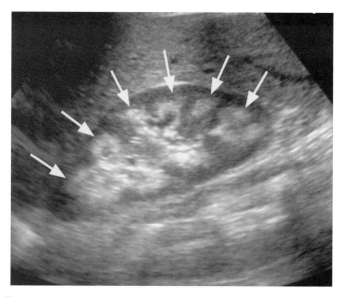

Medullary sponge kidney. Hyperechoic medullary pyramids (arrows) seen in US.

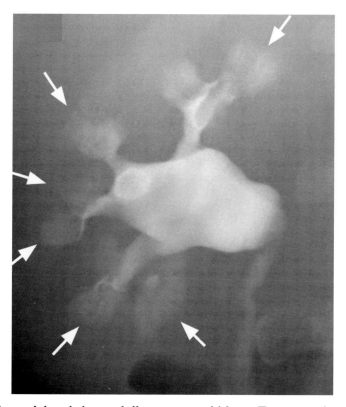

Nephrocalcinosis in medullary sponge kidney. Tomogram from an IVU series. Extensive stippled calcification can be seen within several medullary pyramids (arrows).

Renal developmental anomalies

Horseshoe kidney

- Most common renal fusion anomaly, with an incidence of up to 1%.
- Caused by fusion of lower renal poles in 90% and by upper pole fusion in 10%.
- Associations include:
  - Turner's syndrome.
  - trisomy 18.
  - cardiovascular, CNS, anorectal, genitourinary and musculoskeletal anomalies.
  - vesicoureteric reflux.
  - pelviureteric junction obstruction with secondary hydronephrosis.
- Complications include renal calculi formation and infection, possibly caused by urinary stasis.

Radiological features

- May be imaged with US, IVU, CT or MRI.
- Plain AXR may demonstrate absence of normal renal outlines.
- Long axes of the kidneys are medially orientated.
- Kidneys lie more inferiorly than the normal renal position, at L4/5, lying between the aorta and the inferior mesenteric artery origin.
- The renal pelves point anteriorly.

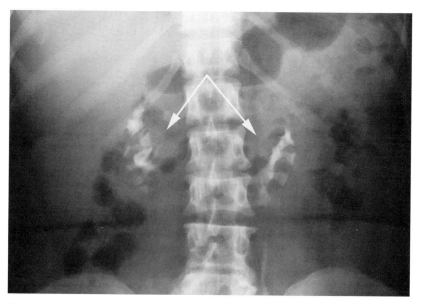

Horseshoe kidney by IVU (arrows).

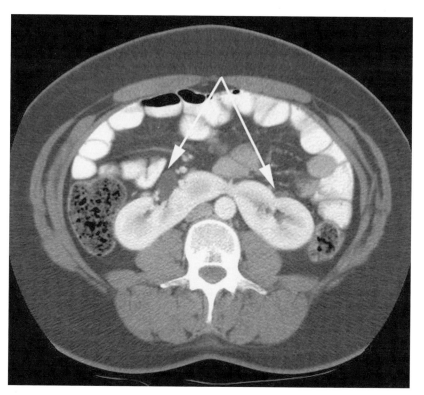

Horseshoe kidney on CT (arrows).

Crossed renal ectopia

- The kidney is located on the opposite side from the insertion of its ureter into the bladder.
- Usually the kidneys are fused (crossed fused renal ectopia).
- The crossed kidney lies more inferiorly.
- Associations include:
  - obstruction.
  - calculi.
  - hypospadias.
  - urethral valves.

Pelvic kidney

- Failure of renal ascent has an incidence of 1:750.
- Often associated with failure of rotation, with the renal pelvis facing anteriorly.
- Associations include:
  - contralateral renal agenesis.
  - hydronephrosis due to a high PUJ.
  - reflux and hypospadias.
- A common cause of 'absent' kidney as seen on USS.

Complete ureteral duplication (duplex kidney)

- Duplex kidney is caused by two, rather than one, ureteral buds arising from the mesonephric duct, resulting in ureteral duplication. Up to 40% are bilateral.
- The lower moiety drains the lower pole and mid-kidney and distally inserts into the trigone of the bladder. This moiety is prone to vesi-coureteric reflux, owing to a short ureteral course through the bladder wall, with an associated risk of secondary chronic pyelonephritis. Pelviureteric junction obstruction is a further complication.

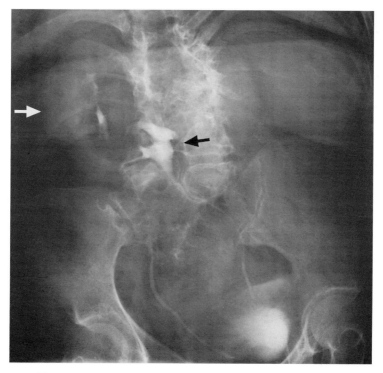

Crossed left renal ectopia. The 'crossed' left kidney lies inferior to the right as seen in IVU, but the left ureter correctly inserts into the left side of the bladder.

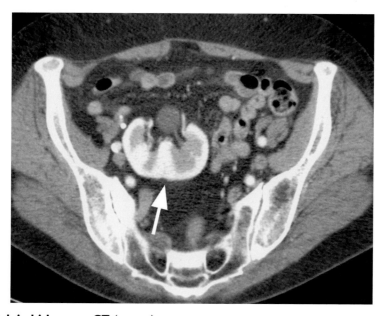

Pelvic kidney on CT (arrow).

- The upper pole moiety's ureter has an ectopic distal insertion, more inferior and medially to the lower pole moiety ureter. In men, the insertion is always proximal to the external sphincter, so enuresis does not occur. It can insert into the seminal vesicles, prostatic urethra and ejaculatory ducts as well as low in the bladder. Men with duplex kidneys are more at risk of epidymo-orchitis. Women with a duplex system may have distal insertion below the external sphincter, leading to enuresis. Sites include the distal urethra, genital tract and rectum.
- In men and women, the upper pole moiety is prone to obstruction because of its ectopic distal insertion. An increased incidence of uretero-coele is seen, further increasing the risk of distal obstruction.

Radiological features

- **IVU:**
  - If both moieties are functional, then the ureteric duplication and the sites of insertion distally will be demonstrated.
  - The upper moiety may opacify poorly owing to obstruction. The associated hydronephrosis may displace the lower moiety calyces inferiorly – 'drooping lily sign'.
  - The lower pole may demonstrate scarring and atrophy, with secondary loss of function through reflux nephropathy. The lower moiety ureter may be tortuous and dilated because of reflux.
- **USS:**
  - The kidney may be enlarged.
  - Two renal pelves separated by renal parenchyma may be seen.
  - Complications such as hydronephrosis or scarring can be identified.

Partial duplex system

- Partial duplex system is a result of a single ureteric bud branching. In distinction to a full duplex system, there is a single distal ureter and bladder insertion.
- It can be associated with obstruction of the lower pole pelviureteric junction.
- 'Yo-yo' reflux, when urine refluxes from lower moiety into upper or visa versa, may occur.
- There is an increased risk of urinary tract infection.

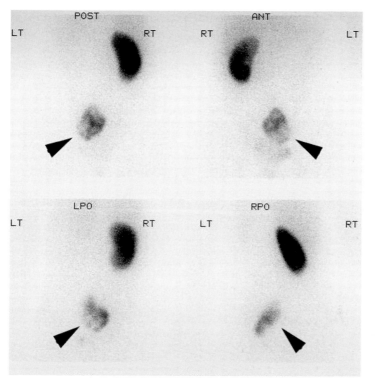

Pelvic kidney. Radioisotope study shows small left pelvic kidney (arrowheads).

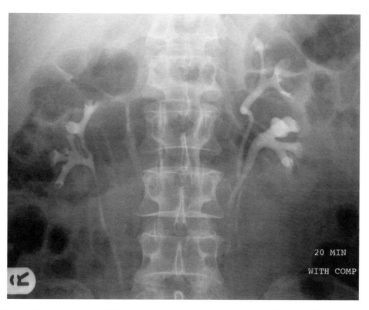

Left duplex system. The lower moiety inserts into the bladder trigone (not shown), whereas the upper moiety ureter usually has an ectopic distal insertion (see text).

Renal agenesis

- If there is failure of induction, the ureteral bud does not lead to formation of metanephric tissue. This results in a blind-ending ureter.
- In formation failure, the ureteral bud does not form, with resultant absent trigone, ureter and kidney.
- Bilateral agenesis, Potter's syndrome, is invariably fatal in the first week of life owing to associated pulmonary hypoplasia.
- Unilateral agenesis is associated with trisomies, Turner's syndrome and Fanconi's anaemia.
- Renal agenesis is associated with other urogenital tract anomalies. In men, there may be agenesis or hypoplasia of the gonads and vas deferens. In women, 40% of patients with renal agenesis have uterine or vaginal anomalies.

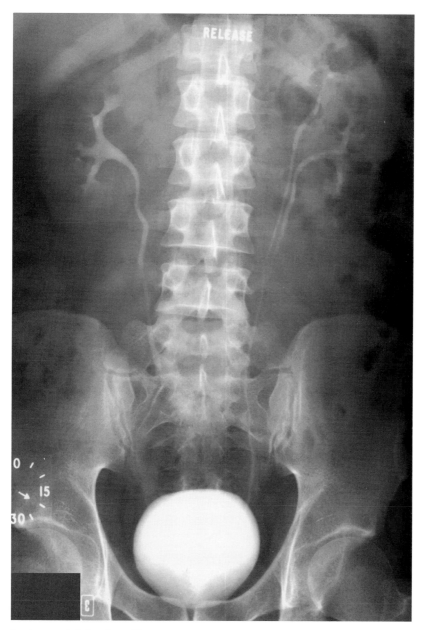

Left partial duplex. The two ureters combine into a single ureter opposite L4.

Renal masses: benign

Simple renal cysts

- The simple cyst is the most common renal mass, possibly caused by tubular blockage.
- In those aged over 50 years, 50% have simple renal cysts.
- These cysts have no malignant potential.

Radiological features

- **USS:**
  - Rounded outline.
  - Smooth, well-defined walls.
  - Anechoic contents with through enhancement.
  - Accuracy of >90%.
- **CT:**
  - Well-defined, thin walls with no enhancement.
  - Fluid density <25 HU.
  - Accuracy of >90%.
- **MRI:**
  - Well-defined lesion of water signal intensity.
  - Low signal on T1W and high on T2W imaging.
  - No solid components and no enhancement.
- **IVU:**
  - Smooth displacement or indentation of collection system.
  - Well-defined defect identified in the nephrogram.
  - Well-defined, non-enhancing exophytic lesion.
  - IVU lacks sensitivity and specificity.

Renal sinus cyst (parapelvic cyst)

- Rounded fluid-filled cyst within the renal pelvis, arising from the renal parenchyma or renal sinus, but not connected to the collecting system.
- Can occasionally cause calyceal obstruction or rarely hydronephrosis. Usually asymptomatic.

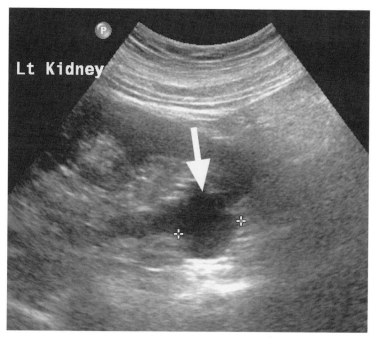

Simple cyst arising from the lower pole of left kidney (arrow). Note the anechoic contents and through transmission.

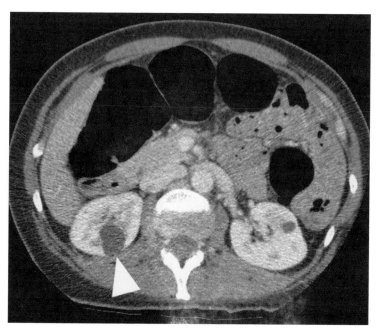

Right renal cyst. Well-defined low-attenuation lesion within the right kidney (arrowhead).

Radiological features

- **USS:** may be mis-diagnosed as hydronephrosis on US.
- On a contrast study, such as an IVU or CT urogram, the lack of contrast within the parapelvic cyst will differentiate it from hydronephrosis.
- If symptomatic, they can be ablated with an ultrasound guided 95% alcohol injection.

Atypical cysts

- Simple cysts may have atypical appearance following haemorrhage or infection.

Radiological features

- **USS:**
  - Rounded lesion but wall may appear thickened.
  - Shifting debris seen within cyst.
  - Internal septations may be identified.
- **CT:** increased density (>25 HU) but no enhancement, owing to increased protein within cyst.
- **MRI:** the usual signal of a simple cyst, low on T1W and high on T2W, is altered, with iso- or hyperintensity seen on T1W, as a result of the increased protein or blood breakdown products. The T2W signal is usually hyperintense but less so than in a simple cyst.

Adult polycystic kidney disease

Clinical characteristics

- Adult polycystic kidney disease is an autosomal dominant condition that results in a collagen defect.
- Carrier frequency is 1:1000.
- Associations include:
  - berry aneurysms.
  - cysts in pancreas, liver and other organs.
  - mitral valve prolapse.
- Presentation usually occurs in the 4th or 5th decade.
- Presents with loin masses, renal failure, hypertension, haematuria, proteinuria and abdominal pain.
- Complications include:
  - renal failure.
  - cyst haemorrhage, a cause of abdominal pain.
  - calculi, often urate.
  - increased incidence of renal cell carcinoma.

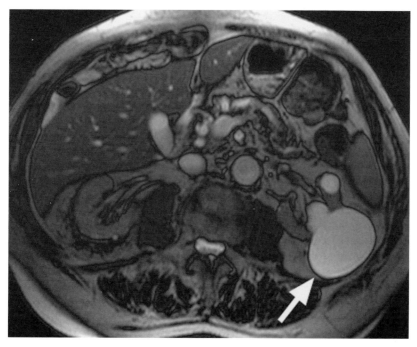

Large left renal cyst. The cyst is of uniform high signal intensity (arrow) on T2W MRI.

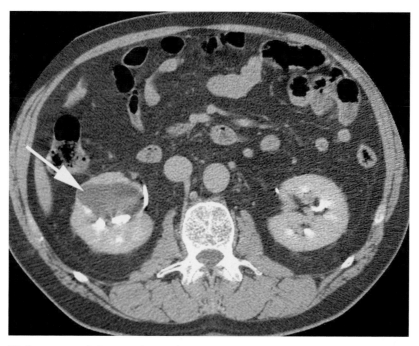

Right parapelvic cyst (arrow).

Radiological features

- **AXR:** not a first-line investigation but may show enlarged renal shadows and curvilinear cyst calcification.
- **USS:**
  - Multiple, bilateral cortical cysts.
  - Enlarged kidneys.
  - Renal outline is indistinct and as disease develops less cortical parenchyma is seen.
  - If complicated by haemorrhage, debris may be seen within the cysts.
- **IVU:**
  - Multiple areas of poor opacification on the nephrographic phase.
  - Distortion of collecting systems.
- **CT and MRI:**
  - Thinned parenchyma.
  - Multiple, thin-walled, cysts. Mural thickening raises possibility of complicating carcinoma.
  - Low attenuation on CT.
  - On MRI, they are low signal on T1W and high on T2W imaging.
  - Following haemorrhage, cyst attenuation increases on CT. On MRI, the T1W signal increases and the T2W signal is variable.

Acquired cystic kidney disease

Clinical characteristics

- Chronic renal cysts develop in patients on haemodialysis.
- There is a 90% incidence after 10 years of haemodialysis.
- Complications and associations include:
  - haemorrhage into the cysts.
  - increased incidence of renal cell carcinomas, with up to 5% of patients developing these.

Radiological features

- The diagnosis is made by the presence of more than three cysts in a patient on haemodialysis, without history of inherited cystic renal disease.
- The kidney will usually be atrophic. The cysts are usually <3 cm, thin walled and will have similar appearances to those seen in polycystic kidney disease, including the findings of intracystic haemorrhage.
- The importance of imaging is to detect developing renal cell carcinomas.

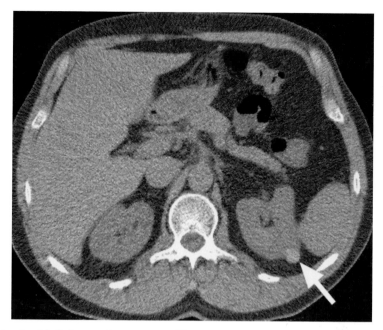

Atypical left hyperdense cyst. The increased density may be caused by haemorrhage or proteinaceous debris.

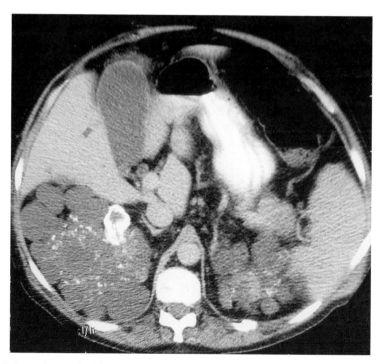

Adult polycystic kidney disease. Multilple thin-walled cysts are seen replacing both kidneys, with no discernible normal parenchyma remaining. Note the multifocal areas of cystic dystrophic calcification.

Angiomyolipomas

Clinical characteristics

- Angiomyolipoma is a benign renal mesenchymal tumour containing fat, smooth muscle and thick-walled blood vessels.
- Incidence is up to 3%.
- The vessels do not have a complete elastic layer, predisposing to aneurysms and haemorrhage. If the tumour is greater than >4cm, there is a 60% chance of haemorrhage.
- Angiomyolipoma is sporadic in 80% and associated with tuberose sclerosis in 20%. There is an association with von Hippel–Lindau syndrome and neurofibromatosis.
- These tumours are often incidental findings, but if haemorrhage occurs, they may present with flank pain or haemodynamic shock.

Radiological features

- The presence of fat within a renal lesion is highly suggestive of angiomyolipoma, although occasionally renal cell carcinoma contains fat, as do renal lipomas and liposarcomas. All these differentials are rare and interval follow-up scans should be considered.
- **USS:** characteristic fat appears as areas of increased echogenicity within a mass, but this is non-specific as calcification can cause confusion.
- **CT:** demonstrates variable amounts of fat within the lesion and may demonstrate the presence of haemorrhage.
- **MRI:** focal fat with high T1W and T2W signal, that show signal loss on fat suppression sequences, is characteristic.

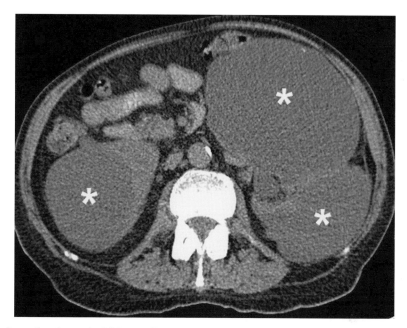

Acquired cystic kidney disease. Large bilateral renal cysts (asterisk).

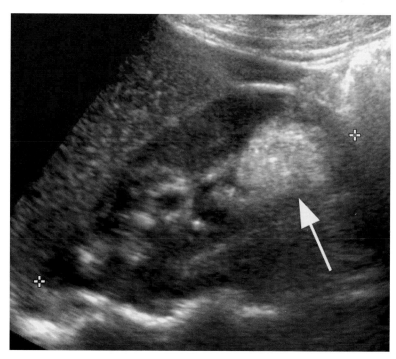

Right angiomyolipoma. Large fatty echogenic mass seen within the lower pole of the right kidney (arrow).

Oncocytomas

Clinical characteristics

- A well-defined tumour seen from the 3rd decade onwards with a peak in the 7th.
- Contains oncoctyes and well-differentiated proximal tubular cells.
- Often has central scar.
- Usually asymptomatic and may be discovered incidentally; it can be up to 10 cm in diameter.
- Unfortunately, neither the radiological findings nor needle biopsy can reliably differentiate oncocytomas from renal cell carcinomas, and resection is usually necessary.

Radiological features

- **USS:**
  - Well-defined mass, often with a hypoechoic central scar.
  - No through enhancement.
- **CT:**
  - Well-defined mass with homogeneous enhancement, but if there is a central scar this will be seen as a stellate, poorly enhancing region.
  - Pseudocapsule may be seen.
- **MRI:**
  - Again a well-defined lesion.
  - The pseudocapsule may be seen as a well-defined low-signal rim.
  - Shows enhancement, although scar may not enhance if present, with peripheral washout.

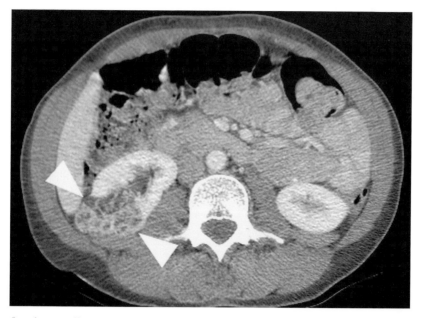

Angiomyolipoma. Bulky heterogeneous mass expanding the upper pole of the right kidney (arrowheads). Note the low-attenuation fatty areas within the tumour.

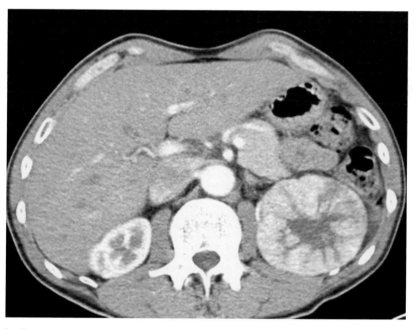

Left oncocytoma. Large enhancing left renal mass with a prominent stellate central scar.

Renal masses: malignant

Renal cell carcinoma

Clinical characteristics

- Adenocarcinoma accounts for 85% of renal malignancies.
- However, 30% are incidental findings during imaging.
- Most commonly present in the 6th or 7th decade; rarely occur in children.
- Presenting features include haematuria, weight loss, fevers, anaemia, flank pain or an abdominal mass.
- Cystic change may occur through necrosis, involvement of preexisting cysts or in the cystadenocarcinoma histological subtype.
- Predisposing factors:
  - von Hippel–Lindau syndrome is associated with multiple renal cell carcinomas, in a younger cohort than usually seen.
  - smoking.
  - haemodialysis (as well as acquired cystic disease of renal failure).
- Metastatic spread includes 'cannon ball' lesions to the lungs, secondary lesions to the liver, adrenal glands and contralateral kidney, lytic skeletal metastases and hypervascular metastases to the brain.
- Direct spread can occur through the capsule into the perinephric fat and the liver.
- Tumour may extend along the renal vein and involve the IVC and right atrium.

Radiological features

- **IVU:**
  - Control film may demonstrate a distorted renal outline and occasional renal calcification. Skeletal metastases may be evident.
  - Following contrast, parenchymal and calyceal distortion may be evident.
  - If there is renal vein obstruction, the affected kidney may not enhance.
  - Generally IVUs are non-specific and, in particular, small tumours may be indistinguishable from other renal masses, such as simple cysts.
- **USS:**
  - Tumours may be hypoechoic, hyperechoic or isoechoic compared with renal parenchyma; most are hyperechoic. Cystic areas may be present.
  - Well-differentiated tumours may appear well demarcated.

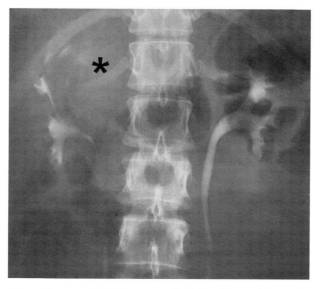

Renal cell carcinoma. IVU shows an ill-defined mass (asterisk) expanding the upper pole of the right kidney with distortion of the upper pole calyces.

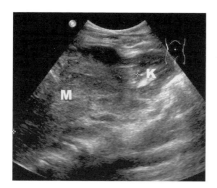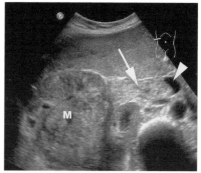

Renal cell carcinoma. Large solid mass (M), seen by US, is replacing the upper two thirds of the kidney (K) with tumour extension (arrow) into IVC (arrowhead).

- Involvement of venous structures (renal vein and IVC) may be seen as soft tissue distending the vessels.
- US is less sensitive than MRI or CECT.
- **CECT:**
  - A three-phase (precontrast, arterial phase contrast and portal phase contrast) CT is usually performed.

- On precontrast studies, the lesion may be homogeneous if <3 cm. They are of increased density (>20 HU) compared with simple cysts. When >3 cm in size, they become increasingly heterogeneous owing to the increased incidence of necrosis. Tumour calcification may be seen.
- Following IV contrast, the tumour generally enhances less avidly than adjacent normal parenchyma, enhancement may be heterogeneous owing to necrosis and cystic elements.
- The boundary between tumour and normal parenchyma is often ill defined.
- The delayed phase of the CECT is very accurate at determining venous involvement; this is seen as low-density filling defects within the renal vein, surrounded by contrast.
- CECT is first-line investigation for tumour staging. It is effective at demonstrating local adenopathy and distant metastases. Direct extension through the capsule into the perinephric space is well demonstrated.
- **MRI:**
  - MRI is the most accurate imaging technique for abdominal staging of renal carcinoma.
  - Renal cell carcinomas are generally hypointense compared with renal parenchyma on T1W and mildly hyperintense on T2W. However, the difference in the signal characteristics between the tumour and parenchyma, on an unenhanced scan, may be small; consequently, as with CECT, three-phase enhancement is required.
  - The 85% of tumours that are hypervascular will show heterogeneous enhancement. Small tumours may demonstrate homogeneous enhancement and may be iso-intense with parenchyma on some phases of enhancement, hence the need for more than one postcontrast phase.
  - The hypovascular carcinomas are usually of the papillary subtype, are often well defined, and on CT can be mistaken for cysts. MRI will demonstrate the solid nature of the lesions, and the presence of subtle areas of enhancement within such lesions is highly suggestive.

Radiological therapies

- There is a growing interest in the use of radiologically guided percutaneous thermal ablation, to debulk or destroy renal cell carcinomas (small tumours) and for patients not fit for conventional surgery.
- Thermal ablation has been performed using radiofrequency probes, laser fibres, high-power focused US and cryotherapy. These can be monitored using CT, US or MRI. MRI has an advantage as changes in temperature affect the T1W relaxation times, which can be utilised to make an accurate, real-time thermal map to assess the extent of thermal injury.

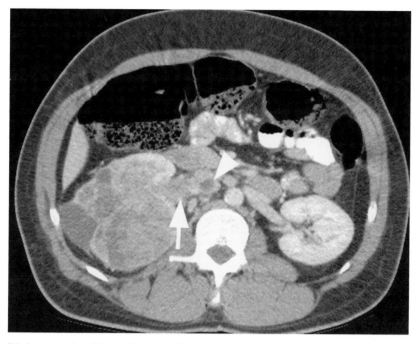

Right renal cell carcinoma. Tumour extends into, and expands, the right renal vein (arrow), with tumour thrombus seen in the IVC (arrowhead).

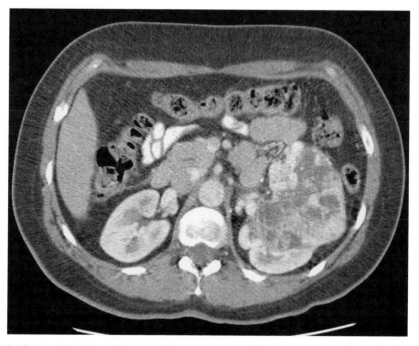

Left renal cell carcinoma. Heterogeneous, hypervascular mass replacing the left kidney.

Renal lymphoma

Clinical characteristics

- Primary renal lymphoma and Hodgkin's lymphoma of the kidney are rare, but secondary renal involvement in NHL is not uncommon, especially in late disease.
- Spread to the kidneys may be by direct extension or haematogenous.
- Presents with a renal mass, haematuria, weight loss and flank pain, but many are asymptomatic. May cause renal impairment.
- Other signs of lymphoma, such as splenomegaly, may be seen.

Radiological features

- Lymphoma is bilateral in 75%.
- Solitary masses in 20%.
- There may be renal enlargement owing to diffuse infiltration but the renal contour is maintained. Renal sinus involvement is common.
- May be perinephric in position, and a kidney surrounded by tumour mass, with no compression or renal function loss, is highly suggestive of lymphoma.
- Renal vessels that remain patent despite being surrounded by tumour are also suggestive.
- **USS:**
  - Focal lymphomatous lesions are generally hypoechoic or anechoic, but without the through enhancement seen in true cysts.
  - Loss of echogenic renal sinus fat is a common finding.
  - General hypoechoic renal enlargement.
  - Other evidence of abdominal lymphoma may be seen.
- **CT:**
  - Single or multiple nodules within the kidneys can be identified. They are of lower density and enhance less avidly than normal renal parenchyma.
  - Other evidence of abdominal or pelvic involvement is seen.
- **MRI:** renal lymphoma is hypointense to renal parenchyma on T1W imaging, and isointense or slightly hypointense on T2W. It shows relatively poor gadolinium enhancement.

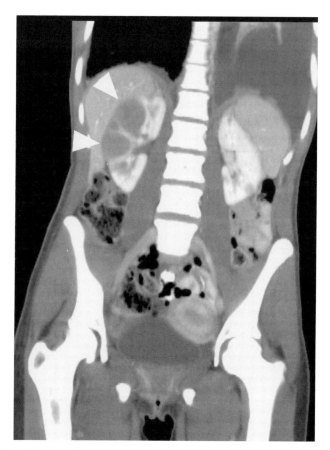

Renal lymphoma. Large, poorly enhancing, low-density lymphomatous deposits within the right kidney (arrowheads) and two smaller lesions within the upper and lower poles of the left.

Metastases to the kidney

Clinical characteristics

- Usually a feature of advanced malignant disease and usually asymptomatic. Does not change management.
- May originate in many types of malignancy but common primaries include lung, breast and GI malignancies.

Radiological features

- Usually bilateral, small, masses in a patient with a known primary.
- May be solitary, especially from colonic carcinoma. Solitary lesions tend to be more infiltrative and less exophytic than renal cell carcinoma.
- If confirmation of diagnosis is clinically necessary, a needle aspiration under CT or US guidance can be performed.

Transitional cell carcinonma

See separate section.

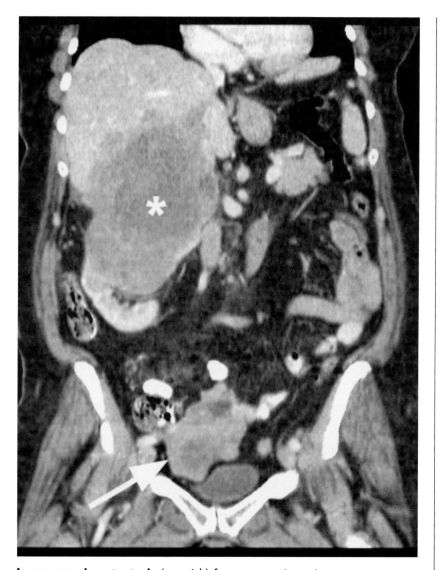

Large renal metastasis (asterisk) from an ovarian primary tumour (arrow). This replaces most of the right kidney and infiltrates into the adjacent liver.

Renal tract calculi

- Calculous disease of the renal tract may affect the kidney, ureter or bladder. It affects men four times as often as women and affects 1–2 per 1000 population in developed countries. The underlying causes are many, with 70–80% of symptomatic patients having an underlying metabolic abnormality.
- Theories as to the pathogenesis include chronically raised levels of calcium excretion, abnormalities in oxalate, cystine, urate and xanthine metabolism, urological sepsis and urinary stagnation, and chronic dehydration.
- Renal calculi may be clearly visible on plain radiography, or non-opaque depending on their mineral content and type.
- Opaque stones include calculi composed of calcium oxalate/phosphate and magnesium ammonium phosphate/calcium phosphate. Poorly opaque stones are composed of cystine while uric acid, xanthine and mucoprotein calculi are non-opaque.
- Calcium-containing calculi either result from a raised level of serum calcium, as in hyperparathyroidism, milk alkali syndrome and sarcoidosis, or occur with normal levels of calcium, as in urinary obstruction, infection, renal tubular acidosis and medullary sponge kidney.
- Similarly, oxalate stones may be associated with primary oxaluria, which is a rare autosomal recessive condition leading to diffuse nephrocalcinosis, vascular calcification, urolithiasis, osteopenia and dense or lucent bands within the metaphyses. Oxalate stones may also form in the presence of abnormal bile acid metabolism, as in patients with small bowel disease, Crohn's disease or large segment small-bowel resection at or near the terminal ileum (site of reabsorption of bile salts in the hepatic–enteric cycle).
- Uric acid stones may form in the presence of chronically raised serum urate, as in gout or myeloproliferative disorders (increased cell breakdown and urate metabolism), particularly during treatment of such conditions. Urate stones may also form in patients with ileostomies or following chronic dehydration (hot climates). Finally, matrix stones are seen in chronically infected kidneys.
- Symptoms, clinical signs and radiological appearances depend to a degree on whether a renal calculus causes incomplete or complete obstruction, or does not obstruct the renal tract.

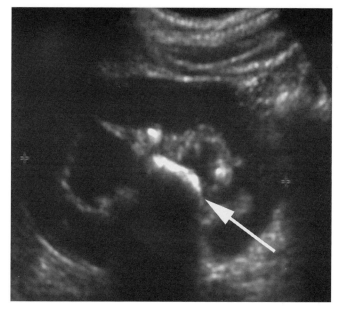

Staghorn calculus within a hydronephrotic right kidney (arrow). Note the posterior acoustic shadowing typical of calculi in general.

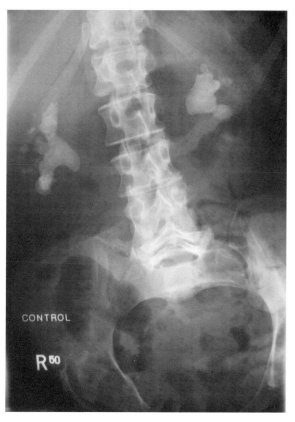

Large bilateral staghorn calculi. Note that this is a 'control' film from an IVU series and not a postcontrast radiograph.

Clinical characteristics

- Renal tract calculi may be entirely asymptomatic. When a calculus causes renal obstruction, this results in severe renal angle pain, typically colicky in nature, radiating from loin to groin, and associated with nausea and vomiting.
- Renal calculi predispose to urinary tract infection. The association of obstruction and infection, unless relieved, rapidly leads to significant irreversible renal damage and may lead to renal failure.

Radiological features

- Plain **AXR:**
  - Radiodense stones may be seen on plain films of the involved area. An important differential within the pelvis is the presence of phleboliths within pelvic venous plexuses. These may cause diagnostic difficulty, particularly in the region of the ureterovesical angles. Hydronephrosis from calculous obstruction may be seen as enlarged soft tissue renal shadows on plain AXR.
- **IVU:**
  - IVU is an important investigative tool in suspected calculous disease. The control film may show radiodensities along the renal tract. After administration of IV contrast, subtotal obstruction leads to a prolonged, delayed, nephrogram and hydronephrosis, the degree of which depends on the degree of obstruction.
  - The site of obstruction may be identified by a standing column of contrast within the ipsilateral ureter above the level involved.
  - In the case of total obstruction, there is, classically, absence of a nephrogram on the affected side with no contrast seen within the collecting system.
  - Occasionally, in cases of total obstruction, high pressure within the renal cortex causes extravasation of contrast within the perinephric tissues.

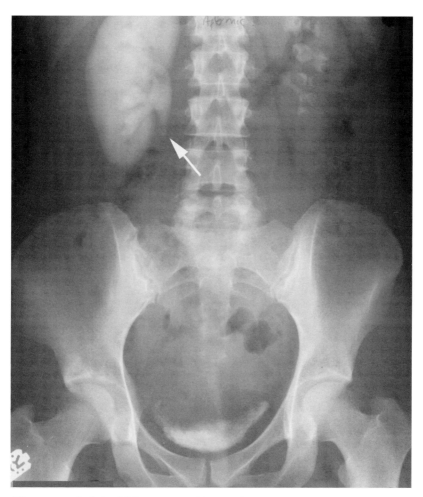

Obstructed right kidney caused by a calculus just beyond the
pelviureteric junction (arrow).

- **USS:**
  - Hydronephrosis is easily identified on US; an important differential is a parapelvic cyst. US may also identify upper and lower ureteric dilatation, although it is less accurate at identifying the mid ureter.
  - Identification of bilateral ureteric jets of urine is important to exclude ureteric obstruction. Calculi may be identified within the bladder as echogenic foci with posterior acoustic shadowing.
- **CT:**
  - NECT is the most accurate method of identifying renal tract calculi; these are seen as radio-opacities surrounded by a cuff of ureteric soft tissue. In contrast to other modalities, CT identifies all types of renal tract calculus, including xanthine- and mucoprotein-containing calculi.
  - CT is particularly useful in identification of small ureteric calculi and may identify ureteric oedema, perinephric stranding and renal enlargement.
  - Following contrast administration, delayed and decreased cortical enhancement of the affected kidney reflects altered vascular dynamics, owing to increased pressure within the distal nephrons.

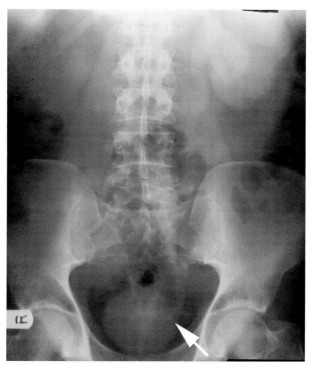

Left renal tract obstruction, with a standing column of contrast, caused by a left vesicoureteric junction calculus (arrow).

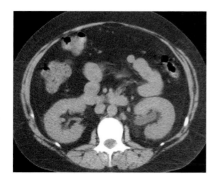 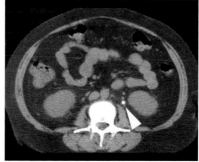

Obstructed left kidney. Renal tract CT shows the left kidney is hydronephrotic. The obstructing calculus is clearly identified, surrounded by a cuff of ureteric wall, within the proximal ureter (arrowhead).

Retroperitoneal fibrosis

- Retroperitoneal fibrosis (RPF) is the pathological formation of dense fibrotic tissue in the retroperiteum, that can lead to complications involving the vasculature, lymphatics and renal tracts.
- Primary RPF (60%) is:
  - probably an autoimmune process, leading to a generalised vasculitis.
  - associated with fibrotic changes in other organs in 10%, including:
    - fibrosing mediastinitis.
    - fibrosing thyroiditis.
    - sclerosing cholangitis.
  - may respond to steroid treatment.
- Secondary RPF (40%); causes include:
  - radiation therapy.
  - desmoplastic responses to great vessel aneurysms or neoplasias.
  - drugs, including beta-blockers and amphetamines.
  - response to retroperitoneal fluid collections.
  - connective tissue disorders.

Clinical characteristics

- Non-specific symptoms such as weight loss, nausea, pyrexia and general malaise.
- Dull pain in the back and abdomen.
- Renal impairment and/or hypertension.
- Lower limb oedema.
- Usually the fibrosis starts at the bifurcation of the aorta and extends proximally to eventually involve the renal hilum. More rarely, it extends distally into the pelvis.

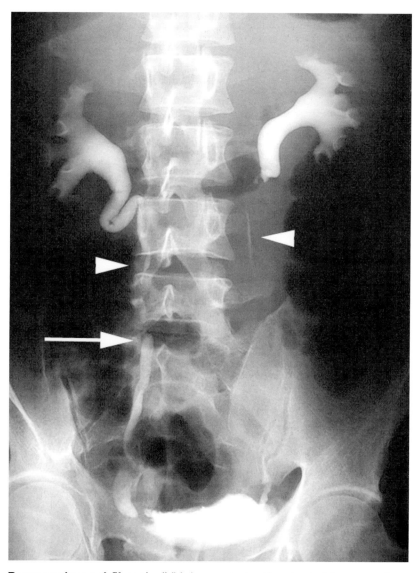

Retroperitoneal fibrosis. IVU demonstrates the classical features of medially 'pulled' ureters (arrow), ureteric tapering (arrowheads) and ureteric ectasia.

Radiological features

- **IVU:**
  - Classical triad of features:
    - bilateral ectasia of the ureters superior to L4/5 from impaired peristalsis.
    - ureters pulled medially by the fibrotic tissue.
    - gradual tapering of the ureters under extrinsic pressure from fibrotic tissue.
  - Generally mild hydronephrosis.
- **USS:**
  - Homogeneous hypoechoic retroperitoneal soft tissue.
  - Renal tract dilation may be seen.
- **CECT:** can show peri–aortic soft tissue, which may enhance if active inflammation is present.
- **MRI:**
  - Low to medium signal intensity in T1W image.
  - May be high intensity in T2W image if there is active inflammation, and low signal if fibrotic.
- **NM:** there is uptake of gallium during active inflammation.

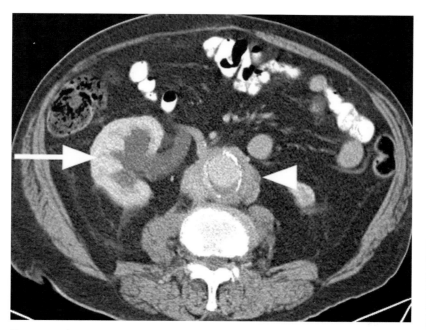

Retroperitoneal fibrosis. CECT demonstrates circumferential soft tissue surrounding the aorta (arrowhead) and encasing the mid ureter (not shown); this results in moderate right hydronephrosis (arrow).

Splenomegaly

- Abnormally enlarged spleen.
- Various methods for assessing size. Most radiologists 'eyeball' spleen for size.
- Inferior tip of spleen extends below the tip of the right lobe of liver.
- Splenic length is longer than 12 cm on transverse diameter.
- Splenic index is most accurate assessment: multiply the three dimensions and a value $> 140\,\text{cm}^3$ is significant.
- In children, the spleen is more than 1.25 times the length of adjacent kidney.
- Spleen longer than 12–14 cm in superior–inferior dimension in an adult.
- Diameter of AP spleen more than two-thirds the abdominal diameter.
- Causes of splenomegaly can be divided according to the degree of splenomegaly they cause.
- **Huge spleen:**
  - malaria.
  - kala azar, leischmaniasis, syphilis.
  - extramedullary haemopoiesis (e.g. myelofibrosis).
  - chronic myeloid leukaemia.
  - lymphoma.
  - Gaucher's disease.
- **Moderately large spleen:**
  - glycogen storage diseases, Gaucher disease, Neimann–Pick disease.
  - haemolytic anaemias, haemochromatosis, sickle cell disease (early on in sequestration crises).
  - portal hypertension, splenic vein thrombosis.
  - causes of huge spleen, in less advanced stages.
  - leukaemia.
- **Borderline splenomegaly:**
  - sarcoidosis.
  - amyloidosis.
  - rheumatoid arthritis (Felty syndrome).
  - systemic lupus erythematosus.
  - haemodialysis.
  - viral infections: hepatitis, glandular fever.
  - bacterial infections: brucellosis, typhoid, tuberculosis, generalised bacterial septicaemia.
  - rickettsial infections: typhus.
  - fungal infections: histoplasmosis.
- Neoplasms of the spleen such as secondaries and angiosarcoma generally replace splenic tissue rather than cause splenomegaly.
- **NB:** sickle cell disease causes splenomegaly early on in the disease, followed by auto-splenectomy following infarction, leading to a small spleen.

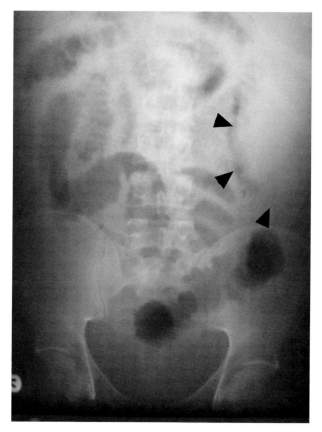

Splenomegaly in a patient with portal hypertension. The lower pole of the spleen (arrowheads) clearly extends below the lower costal margin. Furthermore, there is a generalised 'haze' over the abdomen, caused by ascites, and thickening of valvulae conniventes secondary to fold oedema.

Clinical characteristics

- Splenomegaly can often be detected on clinical examination, if moderate to large.
- May present with dull LUQ pain.
- Presentation is more often with features of the underlying disease process.
- If the spleen is very large, presentation can be with obstructive symptoms such as gastric obstruction or left renal hydronephrosis.
- An enlarged spleen is also at increased risk of infarction and trauma.

Radiological features

- **AXR:**
  - Enlarged spleen is often seen as large soft tissue density mass in the LUQ.
  - Spleen extends downwards and medially towards centre of abdomen.
  - Enlarged spleen may be inferred from displacement of gas–filled small bowel loops.
  - May cause left renal hydronephrosis on IVU.
- **USS:**
  - Imaging modality of choice in initial confirmation of splenomegaly.
  - Usually homogeneous texture on US.
  - Coarse spleen, with similar echo properties to liver in haemochromatosis.
- **CT and MRI:**
  - Splenomegaly is easily identified on both CT and MRI, especially if multiplanar reconstructions are used.
  - Early arterial enhancement of spleen leads to patchy contrast enhancement on CECT and can be mistaken for pathology.
  - Associated pathology is often identified, for example portal varices and cirrhotic liver in portal hypertension or a high–attenuation spleen on NECT in haemochromatosis (from iron deposition).

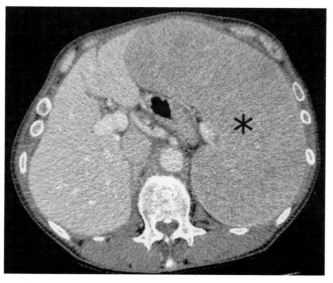

Massive splenomegaly (asterisk) axial CECT.

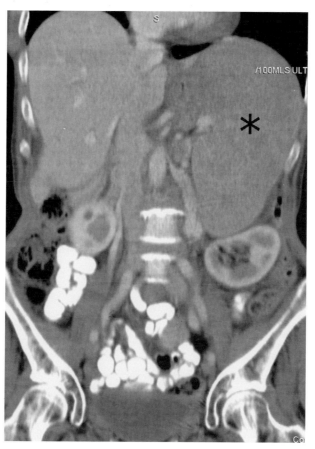

Massive splenomegaly (asterisk) coronal reformat CECT.

Testicular neoplasms

- Testicular neoplasms form 1–2 % of all male cancers.
- Peak age of occurrence is 25–35 years and it is the most common malignancy in age group 15–35 years.
- Risk factors are Caucasian origin, testicular maldescent and positive family history.
- Metastases occur to liver, lung, brain and bones. Nodal metastases are usually unilateral; bilateral in 8%.
- The contralateral testis is at increased risk of developing a metachronous tumour.
- Most (95%) testicular neoplasms are germ cell tumours:
  - seminoma (40%): very radiosensitive with a good prognosis.
  - embryonal carcinoma (10%): more aggressive than seminomas.
  - teratoma (10%): occur in a younger age group (10–20 years) and have good prognosis.
  - choriocarcinoma (1%): most aggressive form.
  - mixed tumours: teratocarcinoma is the most common type; may undergo spontaneous regression.
- Sex cord–stromal tumours are usually benign and hormonally active.
- Metastases: common primary sites include prostate, lung, kidney, GI tract and melanoma. Metastases from prostatic carcinoma account for 75% of bilateral metastases to the testis. Routes of spread include haematogenous, lymphatic, retrograde extension from the vas deferens or direct invasion from an adjacent mass.

Clinical characteristics

- Chronic pain, sensation of heaviness.
- Acute scrotal pain in 10%, from intratumoural haemorrhage.
- Enlarging testicular mass.
- Secondary hormonal effects: gynaecomastia, virilisation.

Radiological features

- **USS:**
  - Sensitivity of 95% for the detection of testicular tumours.
  - Seminomas tend to be hypoechoic; the remainder are heterogeneous in echotexture.
  - Metastases usually present as multiple, bilateral hypoechoic masses.
  - Lymphoma presents as diffuse or multifocal testicular enlargement.
- **CECT:** used for staging the disease.

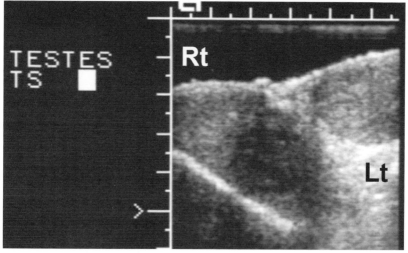

Testicular neoplasm. Well-defined hypoechoic tumour within the right testis. Normal left testis.

Transitional cell carcinoma

Clinical characteristics

- Approximately 85% of urothelial malignancies are transitional cell carcinomas (TCC).
- Risk factors include:
  - smoking.
  - aniline dyes.
  - chronic urinary infection.
  - analgesic abuse.
  - cyclophosphamide therapy.
  - high ingestion of coffee.
- Bladder involvement is much more common than the upper tracts.
- Synchronous and metachronous tumours relatively common.
- Symptoms include haematuria, flank pain and renal colic if obstruction occurs.
- Spread is most commonly to local lymph nodes, the peritoneum or liver.

Radiological features

- Because synchronous tumours are relatively common, the entire renal tract should be investigated radiologically or urologically.

Bladder

Radiological features

- **IVU:** shows irregular filling defect; may have a sessile appearance.
- **CECT and USS:** both demonstrate focal mural thickening and an exophytic mass projecting into the bladder lumen or within a diverticulum.
- **MRI:**
  - Most accurate for staging of bladder TCC.
  - TCC are isointense on T1W sequences and hyperintense on T2W.
  - TCC show early enhancement post-gadolinium injection, allowing accurate assessment of bladder wall involvement.

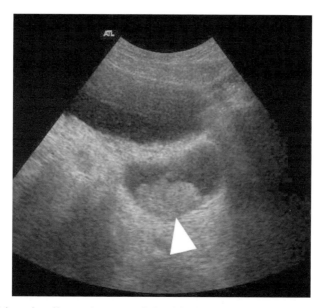

Transitional cell carcinoma of the bladder. US shows solid exophytic carcinoma within a bladder diverticulum (arrowhead).

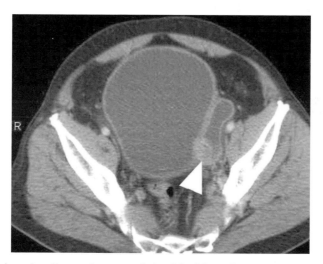

Transitional cell carcinoma of the bladder. Corresponding CT demonstrates the solid enhancing mass within the diverticulum (arrowhead).

Kidneys

Radiological features

- **IVU:**
  - Occasionally punctate calcification may be seen on the control film.
  - Sessile filling defects can be seen within the collecting systems. Contrast trapped within the intersitium of a papilliform tumour gives rise to a stippled appearance.
  - Non-opacification of a calyx occurs when obstructed by tumour. Renal obstruction may be from tumour at the pelviureteric junction. This may result in renal atrophy.
  - Tumour infiltrating the renal parenchyma results in decreased contrast excretion, with preservation of the normal renal outline; this is often not the case in renal cell carcinoma.
- **USS:**
  - Tumour is usually isoechoic or hyperechoic in comparison with renal parenchyma.
  - Depending on tumour location, calyceal dilatation, with or without renal pelvis dilatation, may be seen.
  - Renal infiltration with preservation of renal outline may be seen.
- **CECT:**
  - CT urography is an excretory phase CT of the renal tract and is increasingly replacing IVU. This results in opacification of the pelvicalyceal systems and ureters, allowing assessment of filling defects as in IVU.
  - Mass centred on the collecting system shows variable enhancement. Associated thickening of collecting system wall may be visible.
  - There may be punctuate calcification.
  - Renal infiltration can be demonstrated.
  - CECT is commonly used as a staging study.
- **MRI:**
  - MR urography, either using heavily T2W images, to utilise the hyperintensity of urine, or heavily T1W delayed images, post-gadolinium, can give similar images to IVU but without ionizing radiation.
  - TCC may show heterogeneous gadolinium enhancement, but usually less than the renal parenchyma.

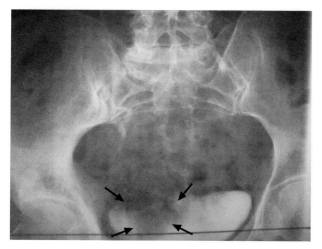

Transitional cell carcinoma of the bladder. Film from an IVU series shows an ill-defined filling defect (arrows) within the bladder secondary to the carcinoma.

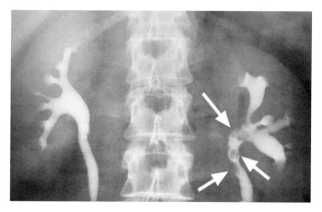

Transitional cell carcinoma of the kidney. Multiple carcinomas create irregular filling defects within the left renal pelvis and upper ureter (arrows).

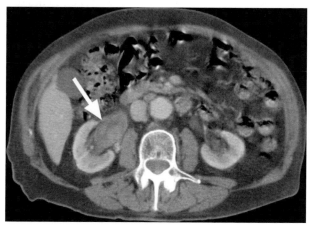

Transitional cell carcinoma of the kidney. Enhancing mass within the right renal pelvis (arrow).

Ureters

Radiological features

- **IVU:**
  - Variable number of irregular intraluminal filling defects can be seen.
  - Irregular luminal stricturing.
  - Variable degrees of obstruction can lead to hydroureter, hydronephrosis or a non-functioning kidney.
- **USS:** may demonstrate features of renal tract obstruction but the ureter, particularly the mid ureter, is often poorly visualised using this modality.
- **CECT:** intraluminal soft tissue mass can be seen. Local extension into periureteric fat and beyond may be demonstrated.
- **MRI:** MR urography can again replicate the IVU findings, but additional sequences are required to stage the tumour.

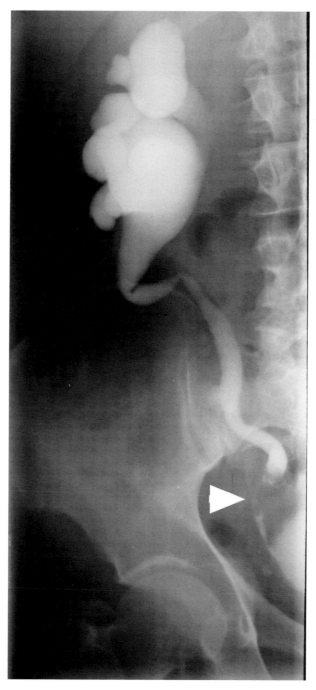

Ureteric transitional cell carcinoma. Obstructing carcinoma of the lower right ureter (arrowhead) with secondary hydronephrosis.

Tuberculosis of the abdomen and pelvis

Clinical characteristics

- Caused by *Mycobacterium tuberculosis*, an acid–alkali-fast bacillus.
- Infections are most commonly pulmonary, but any organ system in the body may be affected.
- Increasing incidence in the developed world as a result of increased immigration from endemic areas and increased numbers of immuno-compromised individuals.
- Presentation depends on affected organ systems. Commonly, there are pulmonary symptoms including chronic cough and haemoptysis.
- Non specific symptoms such as weight loss, fevers and night sweats are characteristic.
- Abdominal symptoms will include the above non-specific signs, with abdominal pain, nausea and vomiting. Urinary tract involvement manifests as non-specific symptoms as well as dysuria, haematuria and sterile pyuria.

Abdominal tuberculous lymphadenopathy

Clinical characteristics

- Multiple lymph node groups are affected simultaneously, most commonly mesenteric and peri-pancreatic groups.
- The main differential is lymphoma, which does not tend to undergo necrosis.

Radiological features

- In 40–70% of patients with lymphadenitis, there are enlarged nodes with hypodense centres and peripheral hyperdense enhancing rims, characteristic, but not pathognomic, of caseous necrosis.
- Other nodal patterns include conglomerate mixed density masses, enlarged homogeneous-density nodes, and an increased number (>3) of normal or mildly enlarged homogeneous nodes.

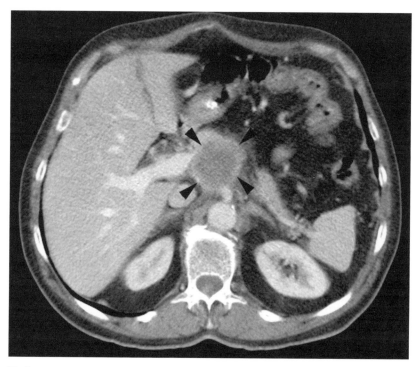

Tubercular lymphadenopathy. Caseous low-attenuation tuberculous node (arrowheads).

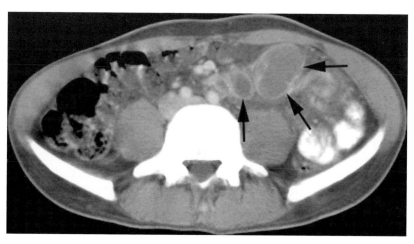

Peritoneal tuberculosis (wet type). This demonstrates cystic loculated fluid collections within the small bowel mesentery (arrows).

Tuberculous peritonitis

Clinical characteristics

- Usually occurs secondary to haematogenous spread or from the rupture of a tuberculous lymph node.

Radiological features

- There are three types.
  - **Wet:** most common, featuring large amounts of free loculated fluid with a high protein density (20–45 HU).
  - **Fibrotic:** large omental and mesenteric cake-like masses with matting of bowel loops.
  - **Dry:** mesenteric thickening, fibrous adhesions and caseous nodules.
- Varying degrees of omental and mesenteric involvement are seen.
- Omentum appears smudged, caked or thickened in equal frequency.
- **CT:** findings in TB peritonitis are non-specific, with disseminated peritoneal malignancy, non-TB peritonitis and mesothelioma as differential diagnoses.
- One complication is small bowel obstruction, and evidence may be seen on imaging.

Gastrointestinal tuberculosis

Clinical characteristics

- TB in the GI tract is rare, but when present usually (90%) involves the ileocaecal region and/or right side of colon. The gastroduodenal regions are affected less often. The oesophagus is the least common GI location affected by TB.

Radiological features

- Skip areas of concentric mural thickening with luminal narrowing, sometimes with proximal dilatation elsewhere in the small bowel, and in the presence of ileocaecal involvement strongly suggests TB.
- Mucosal ulceration is a common feature. Fistulae may occur.
- **CT:**
  - The most common CT finding is mural thickening, which is mostly concentric.
  - Commonly there is focal mural thickening involving the ileocaecal valve and medial aspect of the caecum.
  - Associated evidence of TB, such as necrotic lymphadenitis, may be seen.

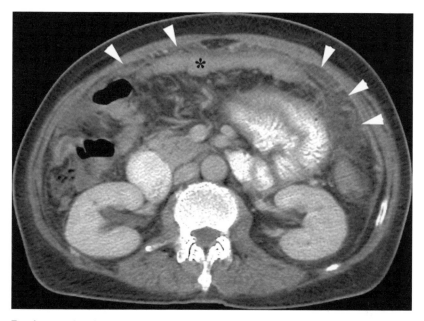

Peritoneal tuberculosis (fibrotic type). Omental caking is demonstrated (arrowheads) with thickening of the underlying small bowel (asterisk).

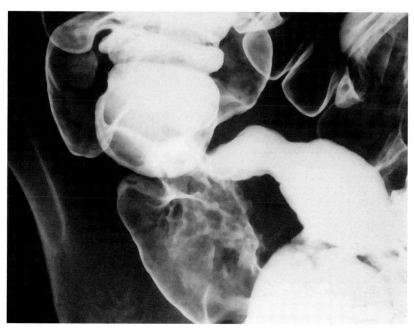

Ileocaecal tuberculosis (barium enema). Marked retraction of the ileocaecal area can be seen, with an incompetent ileocaecal valve.

- **Barium studies:**
  - The terminal ileum may appear rigid with proximal dilatation. The valve itself may be enlarged.
  - The caecum may appear contracted owing to fibrosis and spasm. The affected ileal segments tend to be shorter than those in Crohn's disease and cobble-stoning is not seen in TB.
  - Gastroduodenal TB can result in pyloric stenosis, deep ulceration and rugal hypertrophy as a result of the infiltration.
  - The differential, on barium studies, includes inflammatory bowel disease, lymphoma, carcinoma or other infections.

Hepatosplenic tuberculosis

Clinical characteristics

- Usually caused by haematogenous spread as part of miliary TB.
- Hepatosplenic involvement is categorised as:
- **micronodular** or **miliary:** characterised by innumerable nodules, diameter 0.5–2.0 mm (which may not be detected by CT)
- **macronodular:** associated with tuberculoma dissemination and very rare.

Radiological features

- **CT:**
  - When TB is present, CT shows an enlarged liver and spleen containing multiple non-specific, low-attenuation lesions.
  - The presence of calcified granulomata on CT, in the absence of a known primary tumour, in patients with known risk factors should raise suspicion of TB. Calcified granulomata may represent old, healed TB lesions.

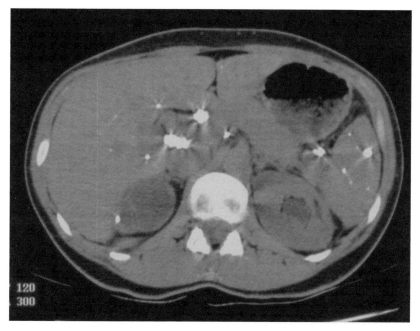

Hepatosplenic tuberculosis. Multiple calcified granulomata are seen within the liver, spleen, portal and peripancreatic nodes. The right kidney is hydronephrotic and a small calculus is seen within the collecting system.

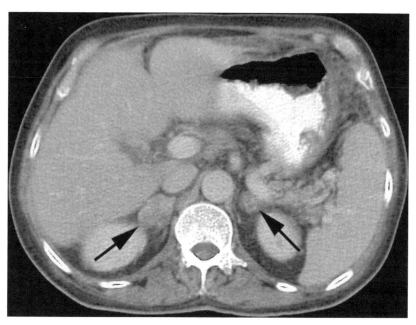

Adrenal tuberculosis. Bilateral adrenal enlargement (arrows).

Adrenal tuberculosis

Clinical characteristics

- Adrenal involvement is seen in up to 6% of patients with active TB.
- These patients almost always present with bilateral adrenal involvement and an Addisonian type clinical picture.

Radiological features

- The CT signs of active tuberculous adrenalitis are enlarged glands associated with large hypodense, necrotic areas, with or without dot-like calcification.
- Old TB lesions can result in dense adrenal calcification visible on CT or AXR.

Genitourinary tuberculosis

Clinical characteristics

- Genitourinary TB is the most common clinical manifestation of extrapulmonary tuberculosis.
- *M. tuberculosis* reaches the prostate, seminal vesicles and, particularly, the kidneys by hematogenous route from the lungs.
- All other genital organs, including the epididymis and bladder, become involved by direct extension of infection.
- Clinical clues include history of TB, sterile pyuria, haematuria, frequency and dysuria.

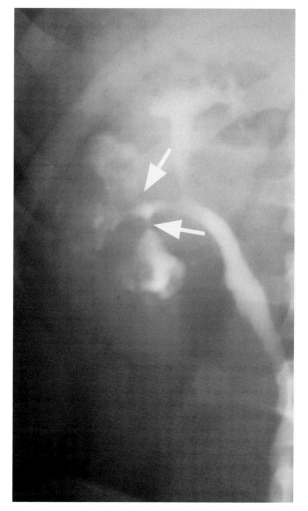

Tuberculosis. (film from IVU series). Infundibular strictures (arrows) within the lower pole of the right kidney, with associated calycectasis.

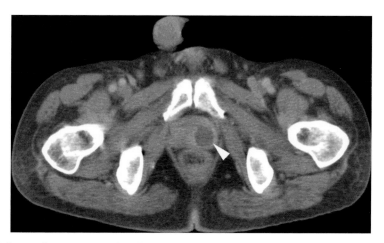

Tuberculous prostatic abscess (arrowhead).

Radiological features

- Renal TB involvement is unilateral in 75%.
- The earliest urographic abnormality is a 'moth-eaten' calyx caused by erosion. It may resemble papillary necrosis but the latter is more often bilateral and symmetrical.
- Renal parenchymal cavitation may be detected as irregular pools of contrast material.
- Dilated calyces with related infundibular stricture at one or more sites within the collecting system may be seen.
- Characteristic calcifications in a lobar distribution are often seen in end-stage TB: known as TB autonephrectomy.
- Ureteric manifestations, characterised by thickened ureteric wall or strictures, occur in almost half of all those with renal TB, involvement being most common in the distal third of the ureter. CT demonstrates focal ureteric mural thickening and inflammatory change in the peri-ureteric fat.
- Sequential bladder involvement is manifested as interstitial cystitis with wall thickening, ulceration and eventual scarring, with long-term loss of cystic volume.
- Genital tract TB almost always involves the fallopian tubes in women, usually causing bilateral salpingitis. Tubo-ovarian abscesses may be seen on US, CT or MRI but are non-specific.
- Male involvement is confined to the seminal vesicles or prostate, which are occasionally calcified.
- CECT shows hypoattenuating prostatic lesions, which likely represent foci of caseous necrosis and inflammation. However non-tuberculous pyogenic prostatic abscesses have a similar CT appearance.

Musculoskeletal tuberculosis

- Musculoskeletal manifestation of TB may be identified. The most common ones are infective discitis and psoas abscesses.

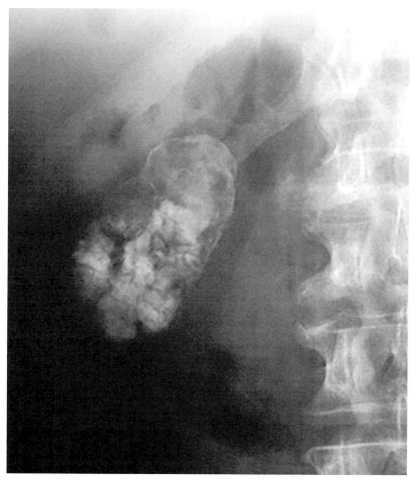

Renal tuberculosis. Intravenous urogram demonstrating a densely calcified, non-enhancing, small right kidney. The appearances are characteristic of long-standing renal tuberculosis; so-called tuberculosis autonephrectomy. The left kidney (not shown) enhances normally.

Uterine fibroids

Clinical characteristics

- Fibroids (uterine leiomyomata) are the most common gynaecological tumour and are present in up to 50% of women over 40 years of age.
- Fibroids are benign tumours composed of smooth muscle and fibrous tissue that are hormone dependent, enlarging during pregnancy and hormone-replacement therapy.
- They usually present well after puberty and shrink after the menopause.
- The clinical presentation depends on the position and size of the fibroids:
  - intramural fibroids are the most common.
  - submucosal fibroids are least common; they lie adjacent to the uterine cavity are most likely to cause symptoms such as menorrrhagia and dysmenorrhoea by enlarging and distorting the uterine cavity.
  - a third, subserosal group, lie on the outer uterine surface.
- Symptoms and complications of fibroids include:
  - pain.
  - abnormal bleeding.
  - torsion of pedunculated subserosal fibroids.
  - subfertility.
  - problems in pregnancy and labour, such as spontaneous abortion, premature and obstructed labour.
  - sarcomatous degeneration of fibroids (rare: < 1%).

Radiological features

- **AXR:**
  - Not a modality of choice, but calcified fibroids may be seen in the pelvis.
  - Circumferential calcification tends to follow pregnancy; punctate calcification is usually postmenopausal.

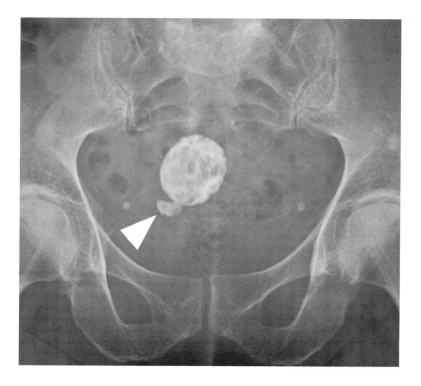

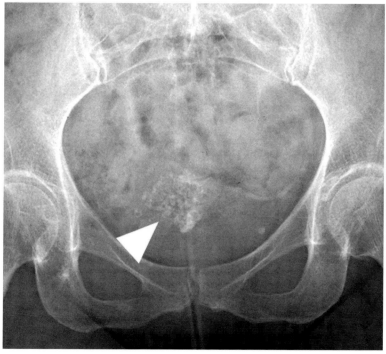

Calcified Fibroids. Two examples within the pelvis (arrowheads).

- **Hysterosalpingogram:**
  - Performed to investigate infertility.
  - Submucosal and larger intramural fibroids will be seen as smooth filling defects outlined by contrast in the inverted triangular-shaped endometrial cavity.
- **USS:**
  - The echogenicity of fibroids is variable on US, with areas of calcification as described above.
  - Fatty, haemorrhagic and cystic areas may also be seen.
  - The uterus can be focally or diffusely enlarged, with individual fibroids measuring a few millimetres to over 20 cm.
  - The uterus may have an irregular outline if there are subserosal fibroids. Large fibroids may compress the ureters, and it is important to check for the presence of hydronephrosis.
- **CT:** not particularly helpful at diagnosing fibroids other than detecting uterine enlargement, as fibroids have the same density and contrast enhancement as the uterine myometrium, unless calcified.
- **MRI:**
  - MRI provides excellent visualisation of the uterus and is used to demonstrate the exact size and location of fibroids, which are of lower signal intensity than the myometrium on T2W sequences.
  - Approximately one-third of fibroids have a high-signal rim on T2W images from peritumoral oedema, lymphatics or veins.
  - Fibroids may degenerate as they enlarge, resulting in heterogeneous signal.
  - Contrast-enhanced MRI is obtained if information is required about the vascular supply of the fibroids, such as prior to uterine artery embolisation (see below).
  - Advantages of MRI are the ability to delineate the relationship of fibroids to the endometrial lining when planning surgery, and to distinguish adenomyosis from fibroids.
  - Adenomyosis is the presence of ectopic endometrium in the myometrium, which causes similar symptoms to fibroids. The diagnosis is made on MRI if the junctional zone (the inner myometrium) is >11 mm thick.

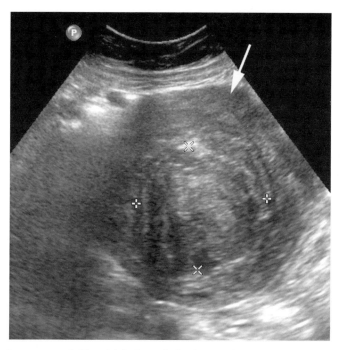

Large intramural fibroid (calipers) displacing the uterine body (arrow).

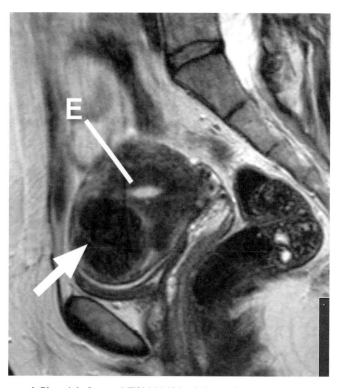

Intramural fibroid. Sagittal T2W MRI of the pelvis demonstrating a hypointense intramural fibroid (arrow). The endometrial cavity (E) is of uniform hyperintensity.

Radiological management

- Medical treatment is only a temporary measure because hormonal manipulation may shrink fibroids but it will not remove them. Hence it is used only in patients awaiting surgery or who are close to the menopause.
- Surgical options include myomectomy and hysterectomy, which can be performed by laparotomy or by operative hysteroscopy. Myomectomy is performed to conserve fertility whereas hysterectomy is the definitive treatment of fibroids.
- Interventional radiological techniques include uterine artery embolisation, where the uterine artery is catheterised via a percutaneous femoral artery approach, and bilateral embolisation of the uterine arteries is performed with polyvinyl alcohol foam particles. Reasons for procedure failure include an aberrant arterial supply to the uterus, incomplete embolisation, very large fibroids or a coexisting disorder such as adenomyosis.
- Newer techniques include MRI-guided focused US and laser ablation, which both use heat to cause tissue necrosis within the fibroids. The former uses thermal heating by US and the latter uses a percutaneous approach to insert laser fibres into the fibroids. In both cases the heating of the fibroid tissue is monitored by detecting changes in MRI sequences to create a real-time thermal map.

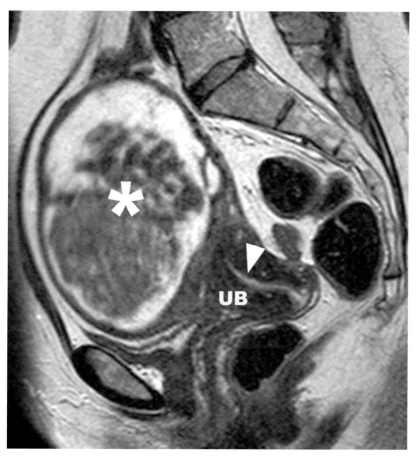

Subserosal fibroid. Sagittal T2W MRI of the pelvis demonstrating a huge degenerate, heterogeneous, subserosal fibroid (asterisk). Arrowhead indicates the endometrial cavity; UB, uterine body.

Volvulus

- Volvulus results from torsion along the mesenteric axis of a segment of the alimentary tract.
- It produces partial or complete intestinal obstruction.
- The ensuing ischaemia results in gangrene and perforation.
- The sigmoid colon is most commonly affected, followed by the caecum, transverse colon and stomach.
- Predisposing factors include redundant bowel loops (e.g. in the chronically constipated), an elongated mesentery, malrotation and chronic colonic distension.

Clinical characteristics

- Colonic volvulus presents with features of bowel obstruction: abdominal pain and distension, vomiting and constipation. In gastric volvulus, there is severe epigastric pain, vigorous attempts to vomit, with little result, and an inability to pass a nasogastric tube.
- The duration, type and severity of symptoms depend upon the location of the obstruction, i.e. location of volvulus.

Gastric volvulus

Clinical characteristics

- Often occurs as a complication of a hiatus hernia
- Two types described:
  - *organo-axial* rotation about a line extending from cardia to pylorus
  - *mesentero-axial* rotation around an axis extending from the lesser to greater curvature.
  - Complications include intramural emphysema and gastric perforation.

Radiological features

- **AXR:** shows massively distended stomach in LUQ.
- **Barium swallow/meal:** shows incomplete or absent passage of contrast into the stomach.

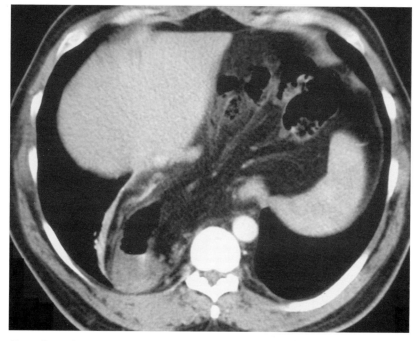

Gastric volvulus. In a large hiatus hernia on CT.

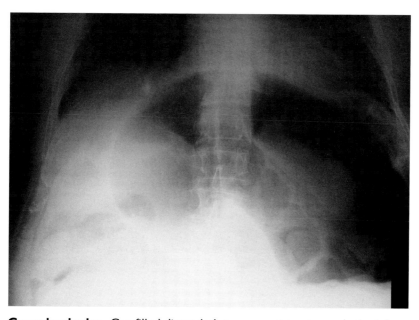

Caecal volvulus. Gas-filled distended caecum rotates towards the left upper quadrant.

Caecal volvulus

Clinical characteristics

- Predisposing factors are malrotation and a congenitally long mesentery.
- Peak age is 20–40 years, more commonly in males.

Radiological features

- **AXR:** 'kidney-shaped' distended caecum rotates centrally towards the LUQ.
- **Instant enema:** the tapered end of the barium column points towards the torsion.

Sigmoid volvulus

Clinical characteristics

- Typically occurs in elderly constipated patients. The sigmoid colon twists on its mesenteric axis.

Radiological features

- **AXR:**
  - Greatly distended loop, with fluid–fluid levels, mainly on the left side, extending towards diaphragm.
  - Produces a typical 'coffee bean sign', with a distinct midline crease, representing the mesenteric root, surrounded by a gaseous distended loop.
  - Associated with proximal bowel obstruction.
- **Instant enema:** 'bird of prey sign': tapered hook-like end can be seen on the barium column.
- **CT:** tightly torted mesentery, produced by twisted afferent and efferent loops, produces the so-called 'swirl sign'.

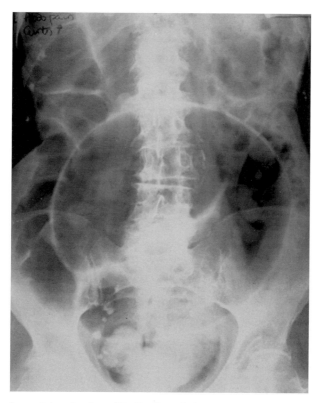

Classic sigmoid volvulus. 'Coffee bean' sign.

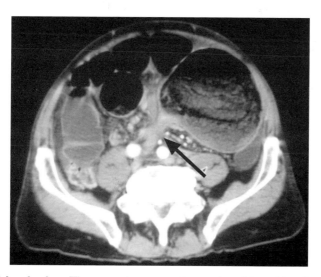

Sigmoid volvulus. The torted segment (arrow) and faecal loading within the proximal dilated sigmoid are clearly demonstrated on CT.

Small-bowel volvulus

Clinical characteristics

- Usually occurs in the ileum and is related to the presence of congenital bands or adhesions.

Radiological features

- **AXR:** proximal small-bowel dilatation is seen.
- **CT:**
  - U-shaped configuration of distended and fluid-filled loops of small bowel converge towards the point of torsion.
  - Tightly twisted mesentery can be seen around the point of torsion ('whirl sign').
  - There are fusiform tapering loops.
  - There may be signs of bowel ischaemia or infarction.

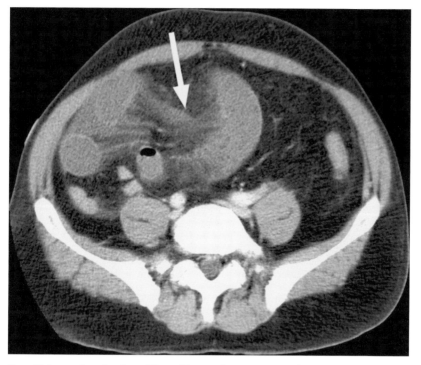

Small-bowel volvulus. Closed loop obstruction and dilated loops converging on the point of torsion (arrow).